You Can Become
A Professional Nurse

Keys to Nursing Success

Pre-Nursing

Nursing School

Passing NCLEX

Beyond Nursing School

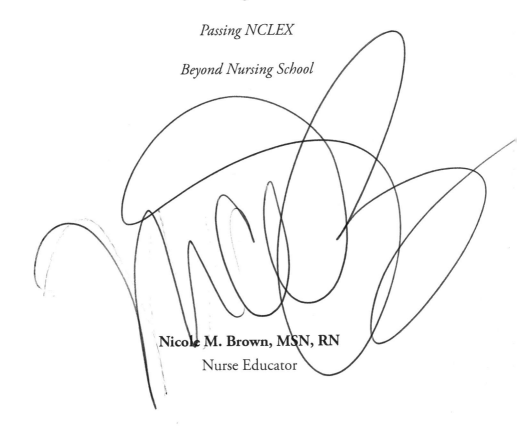

Nicole M. Brown, MSN, RN
Nurse Educator

You Can Become A Professional Nurse

ISBN: Print 978-0-9860963-0-3

ISBN: Workbook 978-0-9860963-1-0

ISBN: EBook 978-0-9860963-2-7

Publisher: Nursing Success College

Layout & Design: Nursing Success College

DEDICATIONS:

This book is dedicated to my three children (Nathaniel, Nicolas & Nicola). Thank you for inspiring me to make the world a better place for you. Thanks to my family, friends and mentors for their support during the process of writing this book. Special thanks go out to my DAD (Jerome H. Brown Sr.) for helping me with everything!

ACKNOWLEDGEMENTS:

I would like to acknowledge and thank all the Professional Nurses who contributed to this project. Thanks for volunteering and sharing your knowledge and wisdom with the next generation of nurses.

A SPECIAL THANKS:

Thanks to all the nursing students who I have taught. I wrote this book because you need information to make the transition to become a successful professional nurse.

SAVING THE BEST FOR LAST:

I would like to thank Joan Wilson Thompson, The Corner Woman, for patience and guidance during the writing of the book and development of the book programs. Thanks so much!!!

Happy Reading to All!!

TABLE OF CONTENTS

WHAT PEOPLE ARE SAYING ABOUT, YOU CAN BECOME A PROFESSIONAL NURSE

"Nursing students, new nurses and experienced professionals can find solutions in this all-inclusive, powerful guide from Nurse Nicole Brown. The personal stories and vast amount of resources make this book a must read."

Elizabeth Scala, MSN/MBA, RN
Author of bestselling *Nursing from Within.*

"Nicole is an incredible role model for our youth to learn about the nursing profession and then once a nurse; to be supported and inspired. With Nursing Success College, Nicole is bringing her talents as a nurse, educator and mentor to the forefront which will serve future generations of nursing success!"

Michelle Podlesni, RN - National Nurses in Business Association (NNBA) President – Founder, Author of *Unconventional Nurse.*

"Considering a career in nursing? Nicole M. Brown will help you prepare for success—and guide you through every step of the journey. Read this book again and again. Keep it under your pillow."

Donna Maheady, ARNP, EdD,
Author of *The Exceptional Nurse: Tales from the trenches of truly resilient nurses working with disabilities.*

"This is a wonderful book. It is written from the heart and soul and easily conveys the challenges and rewards that anyone who desires to become a nurse will face and receive. I have always said nursing is not for everyone, and this book helps the reader get a clear picture of what it's like to make the decision to become a nurse, survive nursing school, challenge the NCLEX and become a nurse."

Kathy Quan, RM BSN PHN, Owner of TheNursingSite.com and TheNursingSiteBlog.com.
Author of: *The Everything New Nurse Book, The New Nurse Handbook & 150 Tips and Tricks for New Nurses.*

"This book is awesome! Valuable information for anyone who is considering nursing as a career!"

Naomi D. Jones RN, MS, CRNI, Founder of Life Coach RN
Co-Author of *Second Chance Living*
Out of the Darkness Into the Light.

"Are you exploring nursing as a career? Search no further than Nurse Nicole M. Brown, whose passion for the profession and our future reaches new levels with <u>You Can Become a Professional Nurse!</u>"

Sharon M. Weinstein, MS, RN, CRNI, FACW, FAAN
Founder of SMW Group, LLC Integrative Health Forum

"This book overs concise, clear and valuable insight from novice nurse to expert, professional nurse and beyond. Highly recommended!!"

Annette Tersigni RN, ERYT- Founder of Yoga Nursing. Author of *The Richest Woman in Babylon and Manhattan.*

"Nicole has put the best minds and resources together in one book. It's the ultimate guide for those seeking and looking to expand their nursing career."

Marsha Battee, RN - Founder, TheBossyNurse.com, Wealth & Wellness LIVE & RN Getaways

"Nicole has done such a comprehensive job in laying out a plan for you to make your dream of becoming a nurse a success. This book is one your will treasure!!"

Cynthia Howard RN, CNC, PhD
Author, *HEAL: Healthy Emotion.*

"Preparation is key and this book certainly provides you with awesome tools needed to be prepared for Nursing School!

You will find great tips from experienced Nurses on any level providing first hand insight on what it takes to successfully complete Nursing school. In addition to receiving the tools for success, you will discover why in our precious field of Nursing the options are limitless. Yes, You Can Become A Professional Nurse and you can help change the world!"

Suprena Hickman, RN, BSN, MBA Founder and CEO - Connecting Women One Escape At A Time.

"Do you have a calling to become a professional nurse? This comprehensive book offers practical advice on getting into nursing school, succeeding in school and then being successful in a nursing career. I particularly enjoyed the Professional Nurse Spotlight sections where the author, Nicole Brown weaves in her own stories and shares her own personal experience of her journey to become a nurse and her career in nursing. This is a must have book for anyone contemplating being a professional nurse."

Lorie A. Brown, R.N., M.N., J.D., Nurse Attorney, President and Founder Brown Law Office, PC and Empowered Nurses LLC

HOW TO USE THIS BOOK

WHAT THIS BOOK CAN DO FOR YOU

This book covers everything about pre-nursing, nursing school, passing National Council Licensure Examination or NCLEX and beyond. It is designed for you to set your long-term professional nursing education goals and focus on activities to achieve your transition from nursing student to a professional nurse.

THE POWER OF PLANNING

The book covers your planning process for your personal goals to start and complete nursing school. In professional nursing school, "you can never be too organized."

PLAN YOUR TRANSITION

Instead of just jumping into nursing school, take time to get your personal house in order. This can be a blueprint to minimize the emotional and physical hardships for you and your family.

FRAMEWORK OF FORTITUDE

Do you have the courage, belief, confidence, persistence, skills, self-disciple, work ethic, self- knowledge and focus to succeed as a nursing student and then as a professional nurse? This book explains the skills you must have or learn to make your dream of becoming a professional nurse a reality.

TURN YOU NOTION INTO KNOWLEDGE

You may have had a "notion" for years that someday you would become a professional nurse. This book will give you the knowledge on how to start, complete and pass the NCLEX exam.

IDENTIFY YOUR STRENGTHS AND WEAKNESSES

Too many students have and will start professional nursing school without knowing what they excel at or need help with. Professional nursing students have limited time and resources. This book will help you identify your strengths and weaknesses which will increase your chances of success.

FOCUS ON FINANCES

Too many professional nursing students do not understand the financial hardships that nursing school can place of them and their families, until it is too late. This book will review financial options that will help professional nursing students be successful while in school.

SOLUTIONS FOR SUCCESS

When you are a professional nursing student, two things can quickly become roadblocks in the pursuit of your education: lack of planning and lack of experience. This book will heighten your awareness of common mistakes that can snare a professional nursing student. Essentially, the principles and keys to succeed in Professional Nursing School are located in this book.

PHASE 1: PRE-NURSING

Before you take the first step of entering Nursing School, there are some things that you need to consider: the schools that you want to enroll in, the school's requirements, time to devote to studying and other details. This first part of the book will talk about the pre-nursing stage.

CHAPTER 1
INTRODUCTION

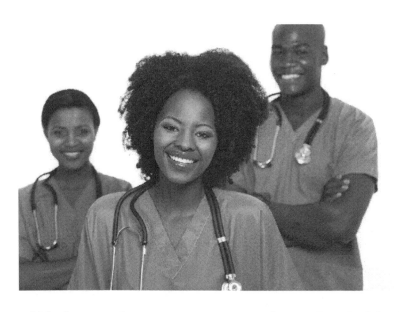

"The biggest adventure you can ever take is to live the life of your dreams." – Oprah Winfrey

Nursing is one of the noble professions in the healthcare field. For so many years, nurses have proven to be invaluable in terms of tending to injured and sick people. In a society without nurses, even the best doctors will not be able to function well within a hospital. Nursing is the largest healthcare profession in the world and voted the most trusted 12 years in a row.

For the reasons stated above, a percentage of the younger and older generations still want to enter this field as a profession. But how does one start their training to be a nurse? First and foremost, you will have to undergo and succeed through the different challenges of Nursing School.

Unlike other courses in a university, this one deals more with practical applications. Students will be trained not only in the classroom, but their skills will also be enhanced when it comes to real life situations. Nurses, after all, will work with real people in their profession. The lives of people are entrusted to nurses! As you embark on your educational journey, this knowledge is ingrained in you.

Nursing school is not the only hurdle that needs to be overcome before becoming a professional nurse – there are the licensure exams that come right after it. This just further proves that becoming a nurse is "not a walk in the park." You have to be certified with all the right qualifications before you can rightly be called a Professional Nurse. It will be a hard road ahead, that is for sure, but when you do complete all the necessary requirements, all the struggles of the years before will definitely be worth it.

This book, entitled, "You Can Become A Professional Nurse," is a guide for those who are interested in tackling nursing as a lifelong profession. This will help you get a background of what nursing school is all about and how it can help with preparing you for the real world. As you go through the chapters, take a serious look at the journey of a nurse in training and may this serve as a helpful reminder for those people who find themselves with a calling to be a successful professional nurse.

TYPES OF TECHNICAL NURSING TRAINING

Certified Nursing Assistant Training (CNA/NA) 6 weeks -1 year training

Licensed Vocational Nurse Training (LPN/LVN) 1 year -18 month training

Types of **Registered Nursing** (RN) Degree Programs that lead to becoming a licensed RN:

Diploma Nurse

Associate Degree in Nursing (ADN)

Bachelor of Science in Nursing (BSN) **(Official Entry into Professional Nursing)**

Types of Advanced **Professional Nursing Degrees** leading to various Nursing Specialties:

Master of Science in Nursing (MSN)

Doctor of Nursing Practice (DNP)

Doctor of Philosophy in Nursing (PhD)

Registered Nurse (RN) classes are typically offered through degree programs in nursing, which are available at the Associate's, Bachelor's and Master's degree levels. RN classes prepare students to meet the needs of patients in doctor's offices, hospitals, hospices and nursing homes.

Programs combine classroom study with practical training in simulated and real-world health care settings to prepare students to pass the certification exam required for Registered Nurses in all states.

Nursing students learn about patient care and monitoring, administering medications, operating medical equipment and working in health care settings. Workplace safety, disease prevention, pharmacology and grief counseling are a few of the subjects encountered in registered nursing classes. A clinical rotation course is also required in all RN programs.

WHICH PROGRAM IS BEST?

Initially, the student has to decide which professional nursing program is for them. Many nursing students start out in a technical nursing training and then progress to a professional nursing degree program. Some people come with a degree in another major and decide to pursue Nursing.

As stated above, there are many options to acquiring a professional nursing degree. If you are responsible, detail-oriented, and have a genuine love of people, you might consider a career as a Registered Nurse (RN). Registered Nurses are vital to our society; chances are you can name at least one nurse who has touched your life in a meaningful way.

PROFESSIONAL NURSE SPOTLIGHT
INTRODUCTION INTO NURSING

When you set your dreams, you must follow your heart. Nursing is the most rewarding career in the health care arena. The passion of caring for others and helping them reach wellness makes my heart skip a beat. If you have a desire to become a Professional Nurse, reach for the stars! The only reason you will never become what your heart desires is simply due to the fact you chose not to. Having a dream is one thing, living your dream is another! My passion to become a nurse started some twenty-six years ago. As a new mother, the news would come that my twin sons had sickle cell disease. As a loving mother to these beautiful babies, it was imperative that a difference was made in their life and the lives of others. This is when my journey started on the path to nursing school. Although there were many challenging times, my heart was passionate about becoming a Registered Nurse. The heart of nursing belongs to those who love caring for people. As you consider your journey into the greatest profession in the universe, please find this quote from Gandhi, "Be the change you wish to see in this world."

Bridget H. Wilson, Ph.D., MSN, APRN Associate Director, Student Health Center Virginia State University
"You can never make the same mistake twice because the second time you make it, it's not a mistake, it's a choice." Author Unknown

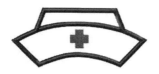

CHAPTER 2:
NURSING AS A CALLING

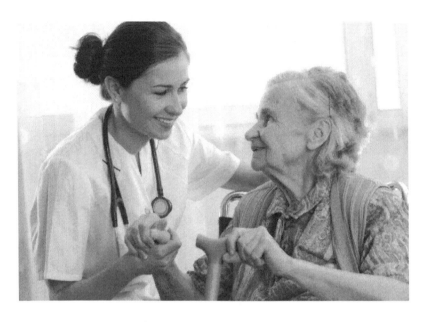

"Constant attention by a good nurse is just as important as a major operation by a surgeon" – Dag Hammarskjold

Nursing is not the sort of profession that you can just go into because of the novelty of being a professional. For business and other creative arts, this might be possible, but when becoming a nurse, you have to have that "calling" for the job.

You will not succeed if you do things halfheartedly. Go ahead and ask professional nurses about their experiences in school and they will tell you that it's not for the weak.

From the first year to the last, you will have to endure pressure and constraints while struggling to learn all about the new concepts that are being established for every lesson. Days on duty at the hospital are not a joke because you will be with real patients who need your help.

However, all of these are merely glimpses of what really goes on in the life of a nurse. The fact that there are so many changes that can happen in a span of a few years, the life of a nursing student might already be a determining factor for some. There are those who started with gusto, but ended up quitting. So before you enroll in a nursing school of your choice, some brainstorming is definitely needed on your behalf. To determine if this is your calling, ask yourself the following questions:

Am I really prepared to be a Nurse?

Can I handle everything that they will throw at me?

Will all the hardships be worth it?

If your answer is yes for all three, then you might actually be nearing that turning point. Ask for some advice from people you know, you have to decide for yourself. Remember that you will be the one taking the classes and it's not going to be easy.

The only ones who are really prepared for this are the people who have decided that Nursing is their calling. When you know Nursing is your calling, it is easy to believe, have confidence, self- discipline and self-knowledge to accomplish your goal of becoming a Professional Nurse.

PROFESSIONAL NURSE SPOTLIGHT
NURSING AS A CALLING

When I was eight years old, my Grandma Ruth was a patient at the Medical College of Virginia Arthritis Clinic in Richmond, VA. My mother, sister and I would drive her from Dinwiddie County to her appointments. The Nurses at the clinic were so kind and compassionate with this older lady with crippling arthritis and I thought, "I want to be like that." My other Grandmother had the opposite experience – she had nurses in nursing for the 8-hour job. They were more rushed and tended to view patients as a statistic or task to be done. I explained to both of my Grandmothers that I wanted to be a Nurse, to help others and fulfill God's plan for me in ministering to the needs of others like Jesus. I told them that my desire was to help others, let my light shine and minister to a person's spiritual, physical and emotional needs. It relates to the teachings of Jesus that I have heard and studied all my life.

My great Grandmother was a Midwife, delivered over 300 babies in Dinwiddie County. My Aunt Ida was a Nurse at Central State Hospital in Petersburg, VA when it was segregated and was the first Mental Institution in the USA for African Americans. I had a cousin that was a Psych Nurse in PA, and one here at Central State Hospital in recent years. Although I come from long line of Nurses, I still felt the calling on my life to help someone that is struggling with illness. I want to help people move toward recovery.

Artrelle L. Spicely, RN-BC Psych/Mental Health Certified Nurse
Central VA Chapter-Black Nurses Association

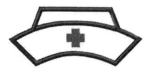

PROFESSIONAL NURSE SPOTLIGHT
NURSING - A DIVINE CALLING

As a youngster, my desire was to become an educator. Teachers were such a knowledgeable and professional group of individuals. I remember sitting in the classroom watching and admiring my teachers and I made up my mind at a young and impressionable age to be just like them.

So, I had it all planned. I would finish high school, go to Virginia State College (now University), graduate with a degree in Education and begin my teaching career. I thought about how proud my parents would be, me being their youngest of six children, the only girl and the only one to finish college. Well, there was one aspect I had not considered; where would the money come from? My Dad was the breadwinner; my Mom was a homemaker, so we were far from "well off."

In my junior year of high school, I went to my guidance counselor to see if grants were available, but the news I received was not at all encouraging. She said even though I was an "A" student, there was no money available for me to attend college. That was indeed a bubble buster. I later learned there were students whose grade average was far less than mine, yet they received grant monies and attended their college of choice.

However, the Counselor did tell me about a licensed practical nurse (LPN) course at the local hospital that I could begin in my senior year where my cost would be one hundred dollars and the school system would fund the rest.

I thought about it for a couple of weeks and decided this was not for me because of my extreme shyness, plus I hated the sight of blood! Then I thought about my work options with only a high school diploma and decided to take my Counselor up on the LPN option.

When I told my parents about it, they were so excited that their baby girl was going to be a Nurse! My Dad went to the local loan company and borrowed the one hundred dollars, had the check made payable to the school and in my senior year I was enrolled in the LPN program.

After graduating from high school, nine months later I graduated from the nursing program and began my "divine calling" in the field of Nursing. I might have thought all of this was by accident, but it was actually by God's design.

In phases within the next thirty years, God allowed me to obtain my BSN, along with my MS and PhD in Health Administration. But in the midst of it all, God called me into Pastoral Ministry. It was then that I discovered how His plan was unfolding in my life.

I have been a Pastor for twenty-two years and I now know that my divine calling in Nursing has best prepared me for my work in Ministry. I am therefore grateful that I accepted the challenge offered by my Guidance Counselor over forty years ago.

At the time I thought I was being snubbed because I was from the "other side of the track", but I now realize that was the best thing she could have done for me.

I recently retired as Director of Health and Counseling Services at Virginia State University and now I am able to truly work in Ministry full time. I continue to have a deep admiration for educators, but my divine calling was to the field of Nursing.

Rev. Dr. Rebecca Branch-Griffin Pastor,
Oak Street AME Zion Church
Retired, Director of Health Services,
Virginia State University

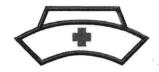

CHAPTER 3: NURSING SCHOOL PRE-REQUISITES

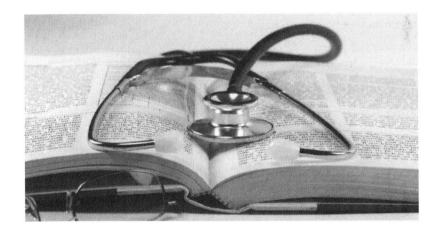

"At the heart of healthcare, we have nurses"
– Donna Wilk Cardillo

Different nursing schools also come with varying prerequisites. Some require more because of their specialized programs. This is the reason why you need to thoroughly check out the requirements of a school, before you apply for admission.

Since Nursing is a part of the healthcare profession, there are some prerequisites that might need to be completed before a student is fully accepted as an enrollee in nursing school. Of course, all the general education subjects have to be completed first.

Primary Prerequisites (Must be completed before the starting most nursing programs.):

- Anatomy & Physiology (A&P)

- Biology

- English

- Math

- Psychology

- Sociology

Secondary Prerequisites (Can be completed while in nursing school, varies with school.):

- Chemistry

- Ethics/Philosophy

- Microbiology

- Nutrition

- Philosophy

- Statistics

- Religion

- Research

The above list provides you an idea of what you, as a nursing student, need to take and pass to ensure a smoother transition into Nursing School. You will also need to provide transcripts to show proof that you have finished and passed the pre-requisites coursework before you are admitted into any Nursing School.

FYI: You must maintain a GPA of 3.0 or better in your pre-requisites to get into most Nursing Schools. So, remember to keep your grades as A's & B's for a chance to be eligible, considered for admission and granted admission into Nursing School. As a student, it is your responsibility to seek help early when experiencing difficulty with classes and in an effort to establish and maintain a GPA of 3.0 or better. Therefore, be proactive in consulting with the instructor, guidance counselor and explore the possibility of acquiring a tutor to successfully pass the required coursework.

CHAPTER 4:
PRE-NURSING TESTS &
APPLICATION

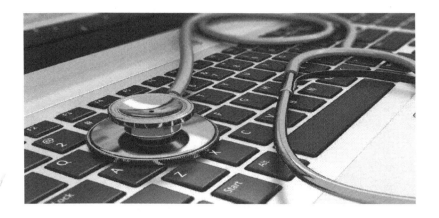

*"When you are a nurse you know that every day
you will touch a life or a life will touch yours"* – Anonymous

You may have found the best school to enroll in; however, typically you will be required to take your desired nursing program's proficiency or placement test (also referenced to as an entrance exam). Now, the name for this might differ from one school to another but the content and general proficiency areas are typically similar in nature. You will be tested for aptitude and qualification; therefore it is advisable that you are well-prepared by allowing adequate time to study before you take the entrance exam.

ENTRANCE EXAM

This test will be mostly composed of topics from your high school years. It's not something that will immediately test you about nursing principles, but it does measure your intellectual capability. It will be a component for the basis of choosing whether you are satisfactory for admission. It will cover the four basic areas of learning, namely Math, English, Science, and Grammar. Don't be scared of this test. As long as you take some time to recall some of your lessons in the last years, you should be fine. There are study guides available for each specific entrance exam into Nursing School. Take time to review them, at least 4-6 weeks before the test.

THE APPLICATION PROCESS

Make sure that you have prepared all the required documents. Some schools do not accept applications that are lacking so it's best to be prepared. Photocopy anything that needs to be duplicated and adhere to all their requirements for admission.

When submitting your applications, do not turn them in too early or too late. Most schools have their own scheduled dates so it is best to go with that so that you don't run into any trouble. Upcoming student applications for the next semester are only processed weeks before it starts, be aware of the schedule for it.

Additional Admission Requirements (Can vary from school to school.):

- Application

- Entrance Exam (Ex. TEAS or HESI)

- Transcripts (Official) from High School and other colleges

- Admissions Essay (Ex. Your Reason to Become a Nurse)

- References (2-3 past employers)

- Background Check (very important)

- Physical & Immunization Records

After you have processed your application, just wait for the letter from the school. Usually, that response should be 30-60 days after the application deadline.

PROFESSIONAL NURSE SPOTLIGHT
PRE-NURSING TESTS AND APPLICATION

Nursing students with disabilities are increasing in number every year. Are you hoping to be one of them? If so, you will need to do some homework and learn about your rights to receive reasonable accommodations. A visit to the campus Office of Students With Disabilities is an important first step. If you will be requesting accommodation, you will need to obtain a letter documenting your disability from your physician, audiologist or psychologist. The Office of Students With Disabilities will require this documentation.

You should also anticipate a wide range of questions related to your disability. Try to rehearse responses to questions such as, "How will you be able to hear heart sounds?" or "How will you be able to lift a patient?" Try to find a mentor and network with nurses and nursing students with similar challenges. Read as much as you can about nursing students with disabilities and join www.ExceptionalNurse.com. The time you invest will be well worth it!

Donna Maheady, ARNP, EdD is founder of the nonprofit organization www.ExceptionalNurse.com and author of "The Exceptional Nurse: Tales from the trenches of truly resilient nurses working with disabilities" and "Leave No Nurse Behind: Nurses working with Disabilities".

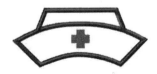

CHAPTER 5:
PRE-NURSING
FINANCING

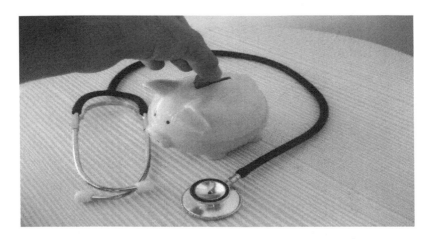

"Education is the most powerful weapon you can use to change the world." - Nelson Mandela

Every student wants to be enrolled in the best schools as much as possible. This is true for all who are looking to study, no matter what the course. But for training and learning for a profession like Nursing, you need to be equipped with the right packets for knowledge and practical application. In short, you need a good school.

THE BEST NURSING SCHOOL

Do you want to enroll in the best Nursing School? Of course you do!

Now, if only it were that easy to choose. The institution that you will be choosing to go to will be responsible for your well-being in the next few years and this is why you cannot simply compromise. You have to choose the best one where you are comfortable. Unfortunately, there is also the question of how you can get in. You might have qualified for the pre-tests and application process, but another big factor that needs to be kept in mind is the tuition fee.

Everyone knows that Nursing is no cheap course. For a period of two to four years, thousands of dollars might have to be allotted for your schooling. Are you able to sustain this?

Choosing a good school is ideal; but take note that most of these schools can also be expensive and not every family can afford to send their student to a top-notch Nursing School with all the good facilities. But do not worry if you are one of these people. As they say, if there is a will, there is a way. There are always options that you can turn to in case you cannot afford to pay the full tuition for a Nursing School.

SCHOLARSHIPS

Like many other university courses, scholarships are also being offered, provided that you have all the right qualifications. These scholarships can be funded either by private organizations or even by the school itself. It's a great opportunity that is presented to the most deserving students who are interested in Nursing as a profession.

But, before anything can be granted to you, there are some requirements that are heavily agreed upon by grantors of scholarships.

You have to show that your grades and GPA are excellent.

You have to pass the interview stage and convince them why you should be the one chosen.

You have to show them that you are an asset for the future.

If these requirements can be met, then among many participants, you will definitely have a greater chance of being selected.

FINANCIAL AID BENEFITS

Grants

Some students may qualify for financial aid in the form of grants. This is free money you do not have to pay back, as long as you pass the courses. Just annually apply for financial aid with the FASFA form.

Work Study

Another method that you can rely on is to inquire about their partial payment schedule. Most schools offer financial aid assistance for their students as long as they provide some volunteer work for the school in return. This is also called a work study assignment.

An application needs to be passed and a screening process will also occur, similar to that of the scholarship process. However, work study only covers the partial tuition amount. This means that you will have to be responsible for paying the remaining balance.

This kind of help is also granted by the school and many partner organizations who aim to help develop the industry with potential assets in the future. Look for institutions that might be willing to assist you with this or approach the Nursing School you have in mind about their policies. Keep track of the details that are needed and work on your application.

Loans

What happens when the other two options are not feasible for you? Turn to student loans. Many countries offer a convenient "study now, pay later" option and you can take advantage of this to help you get through Nursing School.

While it may not be as good of a deal as the two above, this one will also guarantee that you have enough finances to purchase all the books you need and the right equipment to become a Nurse. The only difference is that you will have to pay off your debt in the later years.

CHAPTER 6:
TO WORK OR
NOT TO WORK

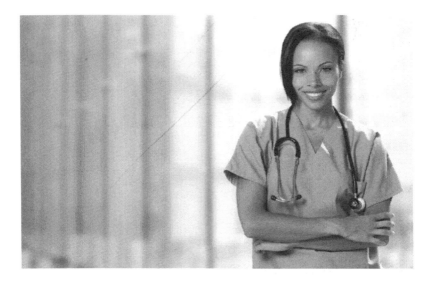

"Nurses are patient people"- Anonymous

Because the nursing courses range on the expensive side, working part-time might be another option that you are thinking of. It's one of ways that you can help lessen the burden of the tuition fees, so it is definitely a viable solution.

But is this really practical?

If you really think about it, being in nursing school and working part-time will really not go together. After all, the course is academic-based and you will end up tired: mind and body. Your part time job will not have any space in this regard and it might only cause you to do things half-heartedly.

If you want, you can always seek out the other options that were listed down in the previous chapter to help alleviate the tuition payments.

Now, I'm not saying that this option is impossible. I am merely pointing out that it is not a good combination to have if you plan to succeed in Nursing School. Once again, it will come down to your priorities.

FYI: Statistics has shown that more nursing students who focus mainly on Nursing School are more successful, than those who work full or part-time jobs. If you must work, work more during times when school is out of session and save your money. Only buy necessities while in school.

PROFESSIONAL NURSE SPOTLIGHT
TO WORK OR NOT TO WORK

The decision to work or not to work was not a hard one. Nursing School takes over your life; in fact, you almost do not have a life outside of Nursing School. I went to LPN nursing 5 days a week, 8 hours a day. It was my only life and studying became my best friend.

Currently, I am going to RN School. Initially, I started the traditional nursing program that was becoming my life again. Then, I withdrew to attend online Nursing School. I work 40 hours a week. Have more time for family and friends. I am engaged, while still pursuing my degree. I guess it depends on the type of program that you attend and your priorities as to whether working and going to school will work for you.

Reverend Sharleece E. Bellagosi Founder:
SE Bellagosi Nursing Agency LPN and RN Student

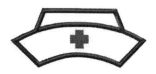

CHAPTER 7:
REAL TALKS -
PERSONAL LIFE

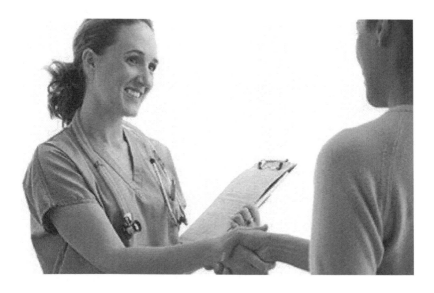

*"As a nurse, every day you know you will touch a life or
a life will touch you"* – unknown

A lot of people wonder about the life of a nurse outside the hospital. Are they as gracious as they appear? Are they like secret agents that live a double life? Well, try talking to a nurse and you might be surprised that they live normal lives.

WHAT IS A NURSE?

A Nurse is someone who cares. They do not just check up on patients and make polite conversations just for the sake of it. They do it because it's their passion to serve. No, they are not the doctor's sidekicks – rather, they are partners. This system allows for the hospital to work like a well-oiled machine.

DO YOU REALLY LIVE A DOUBLE LIFE?

No! Nursing is not like other office jobs. You go in a uniform and work, and after that, you go home. Most staff nurses in a hospital do not have their own office. They have lockers, for their personal belongings. There are some differences, like you have to consider emergency on-call situations or working ridiculous hours which vary from hospital to hospital.

HOW OFTEN DO YOU NEED TO BE AT THE HOSPITAL?

This will depend on the scheduling of the shifts. Sometimes you are needed in the morning, evening or other times at night. It's a matter of knowing who is available and who can work at that time. We all do the same jobs so it's a universal standard that as a Nurse, you will always know your way around the hospital, no matter what the time is.

WILL NURSING SCHOOL TAKE UP MUCH OF MY TIME?

Yes! I was in Nursing School and my personal life was hard. Between studying for lessons and making time for clinical in the hospital, it was a really hard struggle to put everything together. As a nursing student, you will sacrifice your life to learn to save someone else's life. Your personal life will be on hold for a short time. It will be worth it in the end, after you pass the NCLEX and have your first job.

How do you balance all the aspects in life with the profession?

You'll just have to be gutsy enough to overcome everything. Train your body to go with your mindset. Be firm and push yourself as much as you can without actually falling apart. From Nursing School, I had to learn to be tough and it took a lot. But it's an invaluable lesson especially when you are already practicing in the professional world.

WHAT IS THE MAIN INGREDIENT IN YOUR PERSONAL AND PROFESSIONAL LIFE?

Make sure you have a strong spiritual foundation, before entering Nursing School. Accomplish a connection in your personal life with a Higher Power. Having a firm foundation with a Higher Power will be a support system for you, during times of stress in your personal and professional life.

PROFESSIONAL NURSE SPOTLIGHT
REAL TALK - PERSONAL LIFE

What does becoming a Nurse have to do with your personal life? Everything!

Before I became a Nurse, I didn't have a career. I had several jobs that I didn't necessarily like, but they paid the bills. Most of my friends were in similar situations. After training as a Home Health Aide (HHA), I decided that the jobs I had held before were just that jobs. Being a HHA introduced me to the world of healthcare and Nursing in particular. Nursing, as a career, is rewarding mentally, emotionally and spiritually. I saw an opportunity to have a career where I could help people, have a flexible schedule, make a decent salary and have opportunities to grow personally and professionally.

In order to get these benefits, you will need to undergo a major transformation. Once I entered the Nursing Program, I realized quickly that I would have to change some things if I was going to pass my classes and understand what it really took to be a Nurse. Nursing is one of the few professions where you have peoples' lives in the palm your hands.

Unlike many professions, what you don't know (really) can hurt or kill somebody. To be sure you become knowledgeable and skilled in Nursing; you will need to put in the time. As a Nursing Student, this reality affected my personal life in a big way.

Going to Nursing School changes the dynamics of your time and your relationships. As a young mother and student, I enjoyed time with friends and family. One difficult decision I had to make was that "hanging out" with friends and even family had to be re-prioritized.

Real talk is that you will have to make sacrifice's in your personal life. Many people in your circle may not understand your newfound priorities and may intentionally or non-intentionally sabotage your study time. Some may make fun of you for always "being in the books". You will have to let your desire to succeed and your future gains motivate you.

The truth of the matter is when you make a decision to go into Nursing, you will have to make some changes with the people, places and things in your personal life. You may have to leave some people behind. Understanding this concept will help you even when you enter the Nursing workforce.

Because I made the right choices back then, today, I am a Master's prepared Nurse who still loves my profession after over 35 years. The initial sacrifice in my personal life has afforded me a wonderful life. So the real talk about your personal life when entering Nursing School is, you need to get your priorities in order, make the necessary sacrifices and stay determined and focused. You will get your personal life back after school is over along with the benefits from your hard work.

Naomi D. Jones RN, MS, CRNI Founder: The Life Coach RN

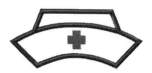

CHAPTER 8:
MINDSET & COPING
WITH STRESS

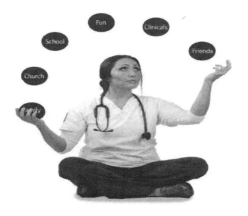

"Nursing isn't a job; it's a passion, it's a part of who you are as a person. And you want nursing students to be sure they have that passion that will intensify for what it is they're coming into in the future." – Unknown

One of the woes of being a Nurse-in-Training is the fact that your schedule will be packed. Between classes and clinicals, there is no time for lingering and daydreaming on useless thoughts. You will need to set priorities because if you don't, your studies can be greatly affected.

BE OPTIMISTIC

From start to finish, it is very important to keep a positive outlook. As a student, you will encounter various situations that will drain all your energy. But do not look at them negatively. Take some time to always reflect about the good things that it can bring you.

You might be bombarded with lessons in your first year, but do know that all of that can be overcome with a happy outlook on life. There are so many things that can help you out in terms of keeping good vibes through the years of Nursing School. You just have to discover them yourself.

Before you start however, try to be open about the things that will be taught. Sure, you might not like some exercises or procedures, but part of being a student is bearing with it. Be optimistic and know that in every hardship that is thrown at you, a silver lining is always present.

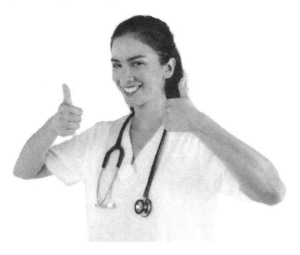

"The essence of nursing is caring" – Jean Watson

CREATE AN ORGANIZED ENVIRONMENT

Make lists, charts, and any aide that you can think of. As long as it helps you compartmentalize your needs, do it. This is one of the best things that Nursing Students can do to help them remember everything. Between the classroom lectures and clinical hours, most students neglect some details and this sets them backward once again.

You have to learn how to take out these items that will affect your productivity. Be organized and jot down everything if you must.

LEARNING TO DEAL WITH STRESS

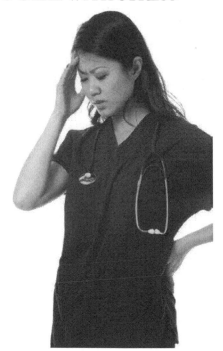

"Nurses can take the pressure" – *Unknown*

Stress is something that will surely creep up on you. In fact, aside from the eventual diploma, this is the only guaranteed thing that you will get from Nursing School. Those eye bags will grow and wrinkles will appear. This is a manifestation of how hard it is to maintain the life of a Nursing Student.

Amidst all this, one has to learn how to cope. Each one is different in their way of dealing with stress and as early as your first year in Nursing School, you have to work on yours. Know what makes you tick and what makes you calm down. Prayer may be the answer, during times of stress while in Nursing School.

Stress is an inevitable factor but as long as you know how to handle it, then it should not pose too much of a threat for your remaining years in school.

PROFESSIONAL NURSE SPOTLIGHT
MINDSET & COPING WITH STRESS

As a future Nurse, your mindset controls your ability to deal wisely with the stressors in your environment – whether they are work, family or home related.

Do you think stress doesn't have an impact on your body, your memory, and your outlook on life?

Check out these statistics:

- The Centers for Disease Control and Prevention estimates that 60% to 70% of all disease and illness is stress-related.

- An estimated 75% to 90% of visits to physicians are stress related.

- According to a study in the Journal of the American Medical Women's Association, 60% of women surveyed said work stress was their biggest problem.

- Job pressures cause more health complaints than any other stressor, says the National Institute for Occupational Safety and Health.

- The 2002 Unscheduled Absence Survey found that while illness (32 percent) is still the leading cause of absences from work, stress (12 percent) was a key factor as well.

I can guess what you're thinking … here's one more thing I have to worry about. We're simply trained to ignore the signs of stress in an attempt to keep the problems at bay. No wonder: changing life-long behaviors is in itself stressful. This is a classic mind-body disconnect.

So, let's begin with mindset. Pretend that we live in a vacuum and that no matter what you attempted, you could not fail. You would only be the very best, achieve the best, and be known as the best. Wow! Is that mindset at its best?

Now, think about what you want your nursing education to be for you. Write out what you would do knowing that you could never fail! If we were to meet at the completion of your Nursing Program, what would you tell me about how your mindset impacted your learning style, your success rate, and your career?

AND NOW, LET'S LOOK AT THE THREE PHASES OF STRESS!

As you know, just being in school today involves stress. Perhaps you are juggling your education, single parenting, and a part-time or full-time job. Here's how most people react to a stressor (such as: earnings announcement, problems at home, manufacturing flaws, countless and mind-numbing meetings):

- First, in what is called the "Alarm Phase", they react to the stressor. This might result in a burst of anger, shock, or surprise.

- Second, they move into the "Resistance Phase," when they begin to adapt to the stressor. They learn to cope with the dysfunction, lack of sleep, or 16-hour workdays. This phase can last for years, and after a while, will feel very "normal."

- Third, the body finally loses steam. They go into the "Exhaustion Phase," where their ability to resist is reduced. They'll feel tired, unable to concentrate, and will often catch colds or become ill – the body's way of slowing them down.

I know from experience that there are many ways to more effectively handle the everyday stressors, as well as those big once-in-awhile stressors. I've taught meditation, mindfulness training, breathing exercises, and disseminated countless bits of information on general nutrition and the benefits of regular exercise.

But, I had no knowledge related to dealing with mindset and stress when I was in my initial Nursing Program. I merely went with the flow, did what I was told, and was resilient. I cannot be there with you when all bedlam breaks loose in your life; I wish that I could hold your hand, provide encouragement, and mentor you personally. But I can state that in times of trouble, the first thing to go – always – is self-care. Nurses are notorious for caring for others at the expense of themselves. Please take the time for you – to renew, to relax, and to restore! Your education and your future depend on it. You will be a better student, a better Nurse/Caregiver, and a better person.

Sharon M. Weinstein, MS, RN, CRNI, FACW, FAAN Founder of SMW Group, LLC Integrative Health Forum

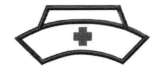

PROFESSIONAL NURSE SPOTLIGHT
COPING WITH STRESS IN NURSING

In the 21st century, job-related stress is a widely accepted phenomenon that demands a significant amount of attention in a variety of industries. From Nursing and Medicine, to Air Traffic Control or Retail, workers face multiple stressors that can negatively impact job satisfaction, work-life balance, as well as mental and physical health.

Those individuals who pursue a career in Nursing are generally caring, compassionate individuals who identify greatly with their role as a caregiver. The culture of the nursing profession can often implicitly or explicitly demand more from a Nurse than he or she is able to give in a healthy or balanced way. With this in mind, individuals must take responsibility for their own self-care and personal boundaries.

Since many nursing programs and employers do not adequately address the management of job-related stress and the prevention of burnout and compassion fatigue, it is in the hands of each nurse to thoughtfully monitor his or her own levels of employment-related stress.

During Nursing School, many students may find themselves pushed to their limit, balancing the responsibilities of home, school, employment, and family. The stressors of Nursing Education are enormous, and the astute nursing student must learn to incorporate positive self-care practices long before entering the profession.

Once employed, the earnest Nurse can actively develop a mindset that underscores work-life balance, clear personal boundaries, and optimal self-care on every level.

MY STORY

Eight years into my nursing career, I began serving as a Nurse Care Manager for a large number of chronically ill, impoverished, inner-city patients through a unique program at a community health center.

Dedicated to the well-being of my patients, I threw myself into my work, bending over backwards to make sure that my patients received the best possible care. I visited patients in their homes, accompanied them to medical appointments, rounded on them when they were hospitalized, and took part in both inpatient and outpatient interdisciplinary team meetings. It was a very professionally gratifying position, but it wore me out on a very deep level.

After four or five years of constant overwork, I found myself experiencing symptoms of burnout, including physical pain, depression, anxiety, and a loss of intimacy and connection with my family and friends. I found myself feeling resentful of my patients, with a decreased level of compassion and empathy, and a worsening attitude towards my work. Meanwhile, I continued to work just as diligently, but with a significantly diminished sense of joy or purpose. It was a vicious cycle, and it took several years to recover my joy, and my sense of personal and professional balance and satisfaction.

PAYING ATTENTION IS KEY

When it comes to your own self-care, and the prevention of stress-related illness and burnout, paying attention is key.

The self-aware Nurse or Nursing Student will regularly monitor his or her own level of well-being, eat well, stay hydrated; practice good sleep hygiene, exercise regularly, maintain healthy boundaries at work, and nurture relationships with loved ones and friends.

A mindset of positive self-care and work-life balance will go a long way towards assuring a healthy relationship between your professional career and the rest of your life.

Nursing is a fulfilling career that offers wonderful opportunities for personal and professional growth, career advancement, and intense satisfaction. However, Nursing can also exact a heavy toll if a Nurse fails to practice excellent self-care on an ongoing basis.

Beginning in Nursing School and your very first position as a Nurse, make sure that self-care and work-life balance are an integral part of your mindset and daily practice. Your nursing career will be better for it, and you will be healthier, happier, and more satisfied, both personally and professionally.

Keith Carlson, RN, BSN, NC-BC
Board Certified Nurse Coach, Nurse Blogger,
Podcaster and Speaker

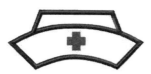

CHAPTER 9:
LETTER OF ACCEPTANCE

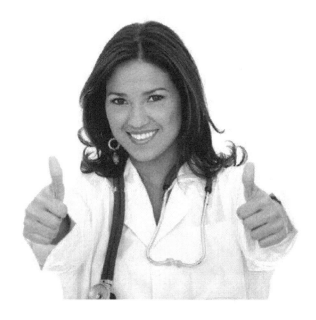

*"I am not telling you it's going to be easy.
I telling you it's going to be worth it"* - Art Williams

WHAT DOES A LETTER OF ACCEPTANCE MEAN?

Much like any other university out there, Nursing Departments also conduct their own entrance interviews and application processes. Depending on where you apply, there are certain requirements that you have to present.

A letter of acceptance is equivalent to an entrance pass for that nursing school. It means that you are qualified and that the institution is willing to work with you and train you into becoming a Nurse someday.

This letter will probably contain some congratulatory remarks from the head of the school and if you applied for scholarships or financial aids, the verdict could be enclosed here as well.

PROFESSIONAL NURSE SPOTLIGHT
LETTER OF ACCEPTANCE

I took several pre-nursing classes in high school to prepare myself for Nursing School. Since I was a child, I truly had a desire to be a Nurse. I did not pursue Nursing for the money. Nursing is a job and a profession that should not be taken lightly. I was determined in high school to keep my grades and attendance up in order to have a better chance at getting accepted into Nursing School.

I remember being persistent with trying to get into a Nursing School. I applied to several Nursing Schools and got accepted into my first choice. I remember waiting for the acceptance letter to come in the mail. Every day, I looked in the mail box and finally it came.

The acceptance letter...what an incredible moment! Congratulations! There is no better feeling than being validated like that. You are now able to embark on that road in pursuit of your dreams with the feeling that others now know that you've got what it takes to succeed.

Enjoy your moment and your acceptance letter, and then get ready for an incredible adventure, future Nurse!

Margarita Jackson, MSN, RN, CCM Nova Southeastern University Nursing Faculty

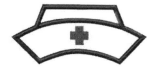

CHAPTER 10:
CULTURE OF NURSING

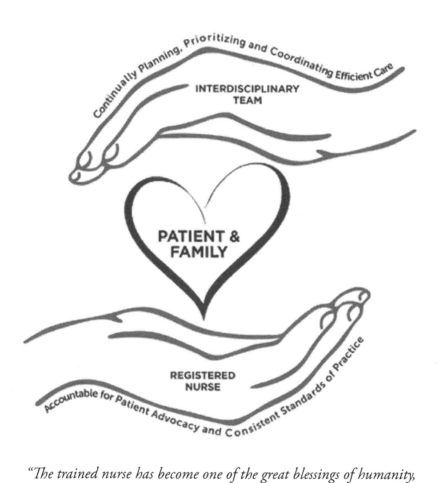

Continually Planning, Prioritizing and Coordinating Efficient Care

INTERDISCIPLINARY
TEAM

PATIENT &
FAMILY

REGISTERED
NURSE

Accountable for Patient Advocacy and Consistent Standards of Practice

"The trained nurse has become one of the great blessings of humanity, taking a place beside the priest and the physician" – William Osler

WHAT DOES IT TAKE TO BE A GOOD NURSE?

This is the age-old question of many people who are interested in entering this profession. But the culture of the nursing profession cannot be defined by mere words. For some people, it is their way of life.

A Nurse knows that his patient is the greatest priority in the hospital. It is their job to take good care of them until they get better. They also need to adhere to certain standards of conduct while they do this.

To be a good professional, one has to be patient, persistent, and prepared. As early as Nursing School, these values are already advocated and practiced by the students.

PATIENCE

A Nurse has to be patient. Simply put, dealing with patients requires patience. Maybe it's just me, but I have always loved these two words that rhyme. In a hospital, they are one and the same. No matter how grumpy, emotional, or irritating your patient may be, a Nurse is there to placate their concerns and get them back to better health.

PERSISTENCE

A Nurse has to be persistent. Yes, even if you are tired, you have to go on. This is probably the motto of most Nurses who are working late shifts over and over again. Unlike stable 9-5 office jobs, nursing does not come with such convenience. Schedules are fickle and they change easily. You might be assigned at early morning shift or you can end up with a evening shift. Either way, you have to persist in keeping up with the hospital operations so that you do not get left behind.

PREPAREDNESS

A Nurse has to be prepared. No matter what happens, alertness is part of the profession. Are all your tools ready? Even the simple habit of bringing a pen everywhere is very helpful in a hospital. For emergency situations, a Nurse has to be calm and clear-minded in order to handle the situation. You might be bombarded with hysterical relatives or bloody patients, but keeping a mindset of preparedness will give you a better outlook for these situations.

KNOW THE HISTORY OF NURSING

This may be a time to take a class on the History of Nursing. The profession of nursing is built on standards and foundations that were led by its history. Pre-nursing students should take the time to find information on the History of Nursing. This will help you stay connected and understand the deep rooted traditions of nursing school and the nursing profession.

CHAPTER 11:
DAILY HABITS &
FUTURE SUCCESS

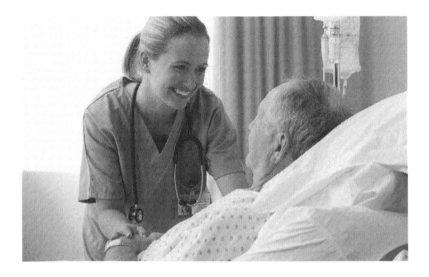

"Nurses know how to prioritize, and how to assess each situation." -
Unknown

There is a really big correlation between these two. Good study habits are proportional to success. This means that before you start Nursing School, you need the right mindset in order to have the ability to cope with the upcoming stress factors that may come your way.

You cannot do the usual procrastinating and cramming sessions that you were so used to back in high school. A lifestyle change might be in order so that you can organize your life efficiently.

Studying will become a part of your life and success will not come easy in this regard. Your future will depend on how you handle things on your end. But these are mere considerations before they eventually materialize. Let's proceed to the next chapter and see what Nursing School is all about and what it has to offer. Know the reasons why you actually need good habits and understand why they will be your strongest weapon for surviving Nursing School.

PROFESSIONAL NURSE SPOTLIGHT
DAILY HABITS AND FUTURE SUCCESS

Working shifts, dealing with some of the most intimate aspects of peoples' lives and managing a multitude of personalities on the job can set up quite a few challenges for nurses. One of the biggest challenges is managing one's own healthy lifestyle! Figuring this out for yourself is going to make your experience of nursing successful along with your level of overall enjoyment.

So many Nurses I know end up feeling chronically tired leading to less satisfaction at home and on the job. Nurses are famous for taking care of others at their own expense. Hidden in the shadows of being a caregiver is the myth that it is selfish to take care of you. Right from the start, recognize that unless you have what you need, you will not be effective in caring for others.

To master your energy, it all boils down to what you eat, what you drink and what you think. Your body is an energy-generating machine provided it gets the nutrients needed. Minerals are the spark plugs of your body's energy machine and this requires eating a diet rich in vegetables. This means having at least half of your plate in color. Eat salads, fresh, steamed, sautéed and juiced vegetables. Have an apple instead of something sweet. Keep your grains to a minimum and eat sweet potatoes or quinoa for your starch. The problem with fast food is it is heavily processed and the ingredients are inferior. It is very high in calories, low in nutrition and it further contributes to fatigue because of the simple carbohydrates and the sugar load. Eat a lean protein with every meal to keep your blood sugar stable and to keep your appetite satisfied.

When you think about food, think about what your body needs for fuel rather than what you want to eat because you are bored. Small decisions add up. If you have a coffee drink every day with crème and sugar you are taking in 300 plus calories and setting up a roller coaster of feeling hyped, crashing, mood swings and irritability. This brings us to what you drink. Water is another energy generator. Most people are dehydrated with the overuse of coffee and sodas that further deplete your body's stockpile of water. Most of the time hunger is actually thirst. Try it next time you feel hungry, drink water instead. Flavor your water with lemon, cucumbers, strawberries or mint to add in some zest. It can also increase fat burning and help you lose weight. Ideally, we need to drink half our body weight in ounces (up to 250 lbs.). Work up to this amount. Your body cannot detox itself unless it has the water on board to flush it out.

The most important part of mastering your energy and your daily habits has to do with what you think. Nursing is definitely filled with stressful moments. In reality, stress has become the new normal today with most people doing more and more and getting less and less from it.

Stress can set up some negative and limiting thoughts. "I do not have enough time," translates into shaving precious time off your sleep so that you go to work tired and end up feeling tired all the time. This new normal snowballs into more negative thoughts.

It doesn't take long for negativity to spiral into bad daily choices and the consequences of poor diet, overuse of caffeine and lack of sleep. This fatigue then can translate into a lack of motivation and the lack of goals and a career that can stall.

Every choice you make should take you closer to your ultimate goal. Choose well.

Cynthia Howard, RN, CNC, PhD is an Executive Coach and has worked with hundreds of nurses and healthcare professionals helping them live and lead more powerfully. www.vibrantradianthealth.com

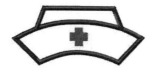

PHASE 2: NURSING SCHOOL – REAL TALK

So now that you have finished with the requirements for pre-nursing, it is finally time to dip your toes in the wonders of Nursing School. For those who are very interested in this field, then it can be said that there will be adventures and surprises that await you in terms of academics and applications.

Being a student nurse will be a struggle – do expect this to happen. There are so many things that you can learn here, and yet, when it comes to real situations, you will still come up short. This is the reason why you should not disregard practical experiences.

They say that school may be about grades, but in Nursing, it's more about being a jack-of-all-trades. Balance is key here!!

CHAPTER 12:
TIME MANAGEMENT

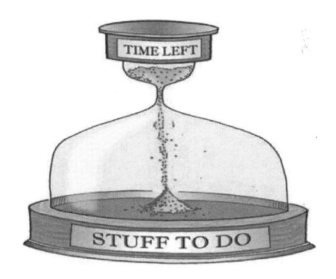

"Nurses dispense comfort, compassion and caring without even a prescription" – Val Saintsbury

When you start your first year in Nursing School, you will already feel the pressures of the course. Basic subjects can be dreadful and confusing, but they are all forced upon that unsuspecting nursing student. This phase can be quite overwhelming because you are still new to the course; but do not be disheartened. As long as you persevere and work hard to pass, there should be no hurdle that you cannot overcome.

THE GREATEST WEAPON

Let us talk about how you can cope with all the needs of this course. What will it really take to survive Nursing School?

The simple answer to that is TIME MANAGEMENT.

Your previous school years will be a walk in the park compared to the experiences that await you in the next two to four years. There are so many topics that you have to keep in mind and procedures that you have to master with precision. Although there is room for error, you need to be fast in recovering from it. This is why you need to manage your time appropriately.

In a battle of wills, time management will be your greatest tool to survive. Compartmentalize everything that you need to do so that you don't end up cramming. Set your priorities straight and get to know what you really need to finish beforehand. Don't be someone who waits for the next day. This behavior will only leave you with double the workload. Believe me when I say that the temporary relief from postponing your work, is not worth the trouble you will now find yourself in.

BE WISE

The ratio of the things to do and the time that you need to do it will probably be not proportional so you have to be able to adapt to this pressure. Instructors might introduce a lesson one day and make you perform a certain procedure the next.

Be someone who is prepared. Read in advance if you have time. This is always better than being the one left behind. Your time in Nursing School is merely a tiny speck compared to the eventual time that you will spend as a Professional Nurse.

This meager two to four years will be the only ones allotted for your training so use them wisely. Make sure that after graduation, you can be someone who is proud to say that you have learned all that you can in Nursing School.

PROFESSIONAL NURSE SPOTLIGHT
TIME MANAGEMENT

Nursing is a demanding career. You need to come each day prepared to work. One of the most important qualities you will need as a Nurse is your time management skill. As a student, learning to manage your time efficiently will help immensely and teach you how to prioritize and re-prioritize on the spot. You need to learn how to plan out your day and stay on track all the while knowing in the back of your mind that things can change on a dime and you must be prepared for the unexpected

In planning out your day, there are two schools of thought: (1) to do the easiest things first, or (2) to start with the things you dread the most. Either way, you have to dig right in and get going. You need to tune out distractions. Put your cell phone away! Make a list of all the tasks so you don't forget anything. See what you can delegate if necessary. (Remember things can change on a dime.) Start with the most immediate need and then cross it off the list. Feel good about your accomplishments as you go along, but don't rest on your laurels; there is still a lot to do. Stay focused!

Try not to be that overachiever and volunteer for more than you can handle effectively. This can translate easily to schoolwork, and basically all of the tasks life throws at you. Be organized and prepared and always ready for the unexpected and you won't be overwhelmed.

By Kathy Quan, RM, BSN, PHN

Founder: TheNursingSite.com and TheNursingSiteBlog.com

Author: The Everything New Nurse Book, The New Nurse Handbook &150 Tips and Tricks for New Nurses

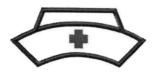

PROFESSIONAL NURSE SPOTLIGHT
TIME MANAGEMENT

As a Nursing Student, you have already proven your tenacity – your ability to apply your skills, hone your performance, and get the job done. But, as a Nursing Student, you are also probably overwhelmed with the amount of paperwork, class time, clinical time, and study. Taking a class on top of work and home obligations is a challenge, and there is a good chance that today's Nursing Student is giving new meaning to the term, "burning the candle at both ends."

The most important skill that you will learn now, and for your future is Time Management. This is the time to speak to your advisor about the course load that you are carrying. This is the time to fine-tune your electronic or paper calendar.

Begin by entering any current commitments at work and at home; then add your class times, homework deadlines, professors' office hours, library house and more. Keep all of this in one place in order to maximize your efficiency – and your time!

Think about what kind of a person you are – morning or night! I had a roommate in Nursing School who was definitely a night owl. When I finished my work and was ready for bed, she was just getting started. She would shower, do her hair, nails and take care of other personal needs. At midnight, the lights would go on and she would start to prepare for the next day's assignments. She was, and still is, a dear friend, but I could not room with her beyond the first year because my body was so sleep-deprived that I could not function. So, think about what kind of a person you are. Plan your study times for your peak periods.

Organize your study materials and workplace. Don't waste valuable time looking for what you misplaced. Break complex tasks down into simple ones that require smaller blocks of time. Don't wait until Sunday night to begin Monday's assignment. Rather, work on it throughout the week and spend Sunday proofreading your materials.

Minimize distractions during study time. If you live at home and have youngsters in the house, take time for your home responsibilities, and then tackle schoolwork when they are in bed.

Some principles of time management from my book, B is for Balance, may prove helpful:

FIND YOUR FOCUS

For one day, notice how often you are not focusing on the task at hand. For example, during a phone call, are you thinking of what you have to do after you are done with the call? Are you straightening the clutter on your desk as you listen to a coworker?

Before you make a call or keep an appointment, take a moment beforehand to say to yourself, "I will give this my full attention." Then do it.

TRACK YOUR TIME

Do you often find yourself at the end of the day wondering where the time went? Consider tracking how long it takes you to do routine tasks so that you can better plan your time.

MAKE AN APPOINTMENT

Right now, make an appointment for lunch or another activity with a friend or relative you have been meaning to spend time with.

ESTABLISHING CLEAR BOUNDARIES

When your classes, work and personal life blend together under the guise of "multi-tasking," then everything suffers. When in class…focus on class. When at work…focus on the job to be done. Make time for your personal life. If you're always talking on the cell phone or checking your e-mail while you're with a friend or family member, your time with that person is not as high quality. Take time to focus exclusively on that person for a while, then you will remember that experience when you're working and you won't feel guilty that you have to concentrate on work.

CREATE A DESIGNATED WORK AREA

If you are a fulltime student in a dorm or apartment, designate your study space. If you are a home-based student, designate a work area for yourself.

SCHEDULE TIME FOR MEALS, RELAXATION AND EXERCISE

You schedule multiple appointments in your personal planner. Schedule time with yourself. Make appointments for regular exercise, a hearty walk, meditation. If you find that you don't have the discipline to keep the appointment with yourself, find a classmate you can include in the healthy activity, and make an appointment with them. You will find that it will be harder to postpone, and you'll have the bonus of quality time with that person.

As a future Nurse, you will impact the lives of many. First, impact your life by managing your time and your responsibilities wisely.

Sharon M. Weinstein, MS, RN, CRNI, FACW, FAAN Founder of SMW Group, LLC Integrative Health Forum

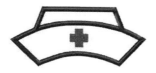

PROFESSIONAL NURSE SPOTLIGHT
TIME MANAGEMENT

When you think of Nursing, what comes to mind? What about nurturer, caring, or smart? How about a giving and compassionate person? Yes, we are all of these things and more. I also like to say dedicated and disciplined. I especially love to say that we work well under pressure. Stress is our middle name and we have to be able to manage it well. So how do you prepare for such a career that is quite demanding of your time and energy? You start by preparing your mind and having an escape plan.

Preparation is key to success and to prevent burnout. There will be instructors that will tell you not to have a life when you begin Nursing School and you should listen to them; however, sometimes it's not so easy, right?

You may have a family to raise with or without assistance, therefore you have to endure the stress of working a full time job while in Nursing School. This doesn't include if there are any family emergencies or unexpected deaths of your loved ones. In Nursing School, you not only have to learn the materials and apply them, but even as a student your actions could potentially cause a death or injury. It will only get more intense beyond school once you obtain your license and begin practicing.

So, do you think you are doomed? Of course not! Remember that preparation is key. You can do this so just follow these steps below:

1. **Effectively Communicate:** Make sure that you communicate with your family, friends, and your boss regarding your educational goals. It is important that they are aware and understand that Nursing School is a priority for you at this time and there will be a huge lifestyle change within you. Don't assume they will know. You know what they say about assumptions.

2. **Establish Your Support System:** Identify your support system. Whether you have children or not, you will need your very own cheerleading squad during Nursing School. Have you heard the old saying that it takes a village to raise a child? Well it takes a village to get through nursing school as well. If you have no friends or family then your fellow classmates will become your friends and family.

3. **Clear Your Plate:** It is important to avoid burnout during this process so make sure you remove anything that would be a hindrance to your success. This includes the rocky on and off again love relationships as well. If you are involved in the community or civic organizations or even church ministries, monitor your time spent in each and decrease accordingly. Nursing School will occupy the majority of your time so make room before you get started.

4. **Get Structured and Stay Committed:** Get a calendar, create a strict schedule, and stick to it! Make sure you place your class schedules, study time (approximately 2 hours/credit hour course), family time, then church and community. It's important to remain balanced and involved, but know your limits by writing it out and committing to it.

5. **Make Time to Escape:** All work and no play will make Nursing Student Jane or Jack a dull person or a sick student. Make time to recharge and get out of the books. Take a walk around a lake, park, or on a beach to detox. If you are an adventurer, then go biking, skiing, or even hiking with friends. It could be as simple as going to a movie once every week or so. If cash is low, then remember the parks and the beaches are free. Take advantage of what Mother Nature has to offer. The serenity is priceless.

You are now armed and ready to conquer Nursing School with success! Just remember that preparation is key to success and preventing burnout.

Suprena Hickman, RN, BSN, MBA
Founder and CEO of Connecting Women One Escape
At A Time

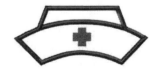

CHAPTER 13:
FINANCES IN
NURSING SCHOOL

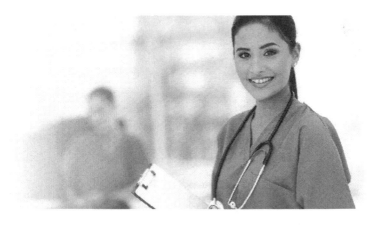

"Nurses – One of the few blessings of being ill"
– Sara Moss-Wolfe

As I have said before, Nursing School is not cheap. For the next two to four years, you might be subjected to thousands of dollars' worth of expenses that will be composed of tuition and other miscellaneous fees. It's a clear problem to those students who are not blessed with a lot of resources.

Choosing the right school might be a factor that can influence the price of Nursing School; but no matter what, you should at least be aware of some details.

Don't be afraid to ask about the assignation of fees for the school's curriculum. Get to know where your money really goes.

Why is tuition in nursing a bit more expensive than the usual college course?

There are significantly a lot more needs for Nursing School students. Unlike other university courses that only require books and writing materials; such is not the case for this course. Since practical applications cover a big part of the curriculum, it is only right that the expenses also follow. A separate pair of uniforms and tools will be used for this purpose and this serves as another added expense for the student.

Here is a list of the most common expenses of students in nursing (tuition and school fees excluded):

- Uniforms

- Stethoscope

- Nursing Kit

- Immunizations

- Books

- Health Check Ups (yearly)

- Drug Screening

The average student spends about $20,000 - $30,000 in Nursing School every year. If you take that amount and combine it with the added expenses, it grows to a staggering amount.

This is the reason why most students opt for financial aid grants or scholarship offerings. Others even go for student loans because they know that the finances in this course are no joke to shoulder.

With thousands of dollars to spend, it doesn't come as a surprise that some families experience a financial decline during the span of these two to four years.

But this expensive price should not deter your motivation to become a Nurse. There are various ways to overcome this problem. You just have to be resourceful enough to go for them.

CHAPTER 14:
MENTORSHIP &
RESOURCES

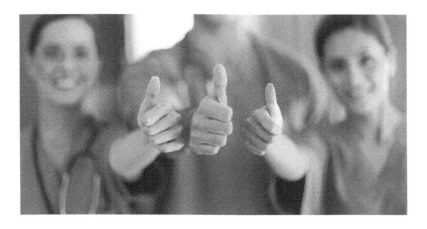

*"Bound by paperwork, short on hands, sleep and energy…
nurses are rarely short on caring"* – Sharon Hudacek

Most instructors in Nursing School are also nursing professionals, so you can be assured that you will encounter some professional working Nurses along the way. They will be your role models and guides as you progress in the next years and what makes them better as teachers is the fact that they work in the field of Nursing.

When it comes to explaining points and experiences, you can be assured that they know all their lessons by heart.

But while you are in school, one thing that you should note down is that you do not have to limit yourself to one medium alone. There are various ways to learn and as a student, it is your prerogative to use them to your advantage. These resources will be a great help in keeping you updated not only with lessons, but also with the latest happenings in the industry.

BOOKS

This is the most basic necessity for learning that you need to have for Nursing School. Books are a basic requirement and you will find that most textbooks for Nursing are all very thick. They cover all kinds of subjects from the first to the last year so this means that you will need to purchase different sets every semester, if it is required.

Despite the expense, these books will be useful all throughout your schooling and even when you decide to take the NCLEX later on.

NURSING MAGAZINES

These magazines will be your gateway to learning about the latest updates in the Nursing and Medical field. You can learn about the latest discoveries, and of course, some of the choice careers that you can go for. It will be a helpful guide in getting to know the industry and your eventual work environment.

MENTORS

For practical applications, you know that you cannot rely on books alone. Seek out personal Nursing Mentors and ask for advice about the best course of action that you can take for some practical procedures.

Don't be afraid to speak you mind. Ask about the things that you are not sure about. This will enable you to perform better as you progress through the years.

PROFESSIONAL NURSE SPOTLIGHT
MENTORSHIP & RESOURCES

If we want to be successful in our nursing careers; we need to find Nurses that are successful and model them. When I first started Nursing I thought that I would like to work with post op surgical patients. So while I was still in school, I asked if I could observe in the surgical ICU. I was able to see for sure if this environment was one that I wanted and at the same time I met many of the Nurses that ended up being my co-workers. I let the Nurse-In-Charge know that I was interested in learning and asked if she would give me pointers. She acted in the role of a mentor even before I graduated.

I definitely attribute my success to having great role models and mentors. In fact, I would have never been able to become an executive for several large companies if it were not for a Nurse that was my boss very early on in my career. Rhonda Crowley was the Director of Georgia Medical Care Foundation and she gave me my first opportunity to be a manager. I made several mistakes managing people and one day, a very big one.

Instead of firing or demoting me, she took me in her office and shared with me what I should be doing. She did it in such a way as to encourage as well as educate me. I am forever grateful to her for the time, interest and the manner in which she was guiding me.

As I rose through the ranks, I had wonderful non-nurses that were mentors too. I learned there is a business side to business and how important certain numbers and metrics were. When I decided to write a book to share with other Nurses the ways in which to reinvent their careers, I had a book mentor that called me every couple of weeks to see what progress I had made. There are all kinds of mentors, role models and resources out there.

The biggest thing is to ask for help. Now, in my role as the President of the National Nurses in Business Association, I have the opportunity to encourage Nurse Entrepreneurship - to educate and connect Nurses from all over the country to succeed in Business.

Becoming a Nurse is a rewarding and exciting adventure. The opportunities out there are limitless!

Michelle Podlesni Business Coach and Bestselling Author
Founder of the Unconventional Nurse

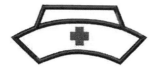

CHAPTER 15: LECTURE/CLASSROOM

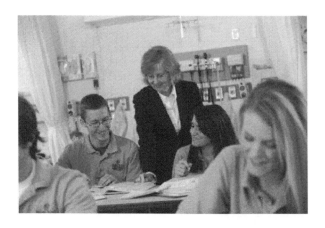

"If love can't cure it, nurses can" – Anonymous

Lectures make up one-half of the curriculum for Nursing Schools. All throughout the semesters, you can expect that this will still be a part of your life. All those nursing concepts need to be learned and in order for you to absorb them efficiently, you will have to work on your ability to focus. Instructors who know their parts relay these lessons and you can be sure that they will not be easy on you even if this is your first year in Nursing School.

The topics can range from general science subjects to practical applications.

Some Nursing Schools offer alternate schedules for their students so that they have lectures first, then practice lab will be next. This allows them to put the lectures into practice that were previously discussed.

Depending on their teaching style, you might have to find your own way of coping and catching up for every lesson that they impart. Unlike high school classes, expect that you will not be spoon-fed. You will eventually realize that the process of learning through these lectures will ultimately be associated with your motivation to study.

Here is a list of the most common subjects that are given as lectures in the two to four years of Nursing School:

- Communication

- Health Assessment

- Nursing Technology

- Nursing Care for the Elderly

- Role Development in Nursing

- Patient Care

- Psychiatric Nursing

- Pathophysiology

- Pharmacology

- Adult Health

- Child Health

- Public Health

- Research

- Caring For Pregnant Women

- Critical Patients Care

- Oncology

- Emergency Nursing

- Practicing Safety in Clinical Practice

- Breastfeeding

- Laws and Ethics for the Health Care Professional

- Forensic Nursing

- Alternative Medicine in Health Care

- Nursing History

- Philosophical, Theoretical, and Ethical Basis for Nursing

- Surgical Procedure Assistance

- Pediatrics

- Women's Health

- Teaching Strategies in Nursing

- Disease Prevention

- Illness Management

- Diagnostics and Therapeutics

- Diagnosis of Mental Disorders

- Psychotherapeutic Modalities

- Leadership in Health Care

- Management of Health Systems

- AIDS Care

- Health Disparities in Practice

- School Health

- Clinical Simulations

- Advanced Research

- Violence Research

- Stress Management

- Cardiovascular Health

- Responsibilities of a Nurse

- Health Economics

- Information Technology and Nursing

The list above is nothing definite. These are merely the general topics covered by some of the lectures in Nursing School. For most instructors, it will also depend on their approach to a topic. There are also variations of the curriculums offered from one school to another. Basically, the lectures will be comparable to how the whole thing is structured by the school.

PROFESSIONAL NURSE SPOTLIGHT
THE NURSING LECTURE/CLASSROOM

The nursing lecture is the format most Nursing Schools will use to provide instruction. Through this information sharing venue, instructors will serve as facilitators of knowledge. Most instruction will use a lecture/discussion format. It will be very important for the nursing student to read before attending class. Typically, on the first day of class, the instructor will present a detailed syllabus with course outcomes/goals and objectives each student will need to obtain by the end of the semester. Along with the syllabus will be a calendar with the reading schedule, test schedule, quizzes and special assignments.

Course expectations are clear and students must adhere to the schedule of activities. The students will receive a study guide to help assist with student success of the lecture material. All students enrolled in the course must purchase the required textbooks and learning resources. Mastery at a minimum level for success will be essential. Generally, students cannot progress to the next course without satisfactorily completing the previous course.

Information presented during lectures will be presented in modules. These modules will be introduced in the syllabus and will identify the concepts to be discussed in class. Each module will build upon the previous one. Studying and coming to class prepared is a must. Although you are an adult, the expectations are for to attend lectures on a regular basis. Catching up is very difficult in that a great deal of information is covered in each module.

The nursing lecture will provide the foundation for the clinical rotation. The lecture which is generally cognitive in nature will introduce psychomotor concepts essential for clinical performance. Students will receive evidenced based instruction on concepts important to safe and effective nursing care. Students will have the opportunity to practice the skills prior to direct patient contact.

The lecture group will meet for class three to six hours weekly. This consists of class time or didactic instruction and laboratory time in preparation for clinical rotations in the healthcare settings. Nursing education requires the acquisition of cognitive, psychomotor, and affective abilities. This is essential to the art and science of professional nursing. Acquiring these abilities start with the nursing lecture.

Karen Faison, APRN, PhD, CNE
Former, Director of Department of Nursing, Virginia State University, Member -Virginia Nurses Association & Central VA Chapter - Black Nurses Association

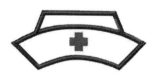

CHAPTER 16:
CLINICAL /PRACTICE LAB

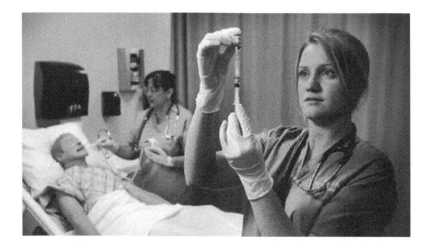

"What happens in clinical, stays in clinical" – Unknown

On the other side of the spectrum, there is the clinical side of things. **The practice laboratory allows the student to practice the skills, before going to the hospital to perform clinical procedures.** This is very important for nursing students because in their hospital work environment later on, they won't be able to function if all they know about are concepts and theories learned in lecture.

By incorporating these laboratory subjects together with the lectures, students are able to effectively implement what they have learned during those times.

As a Nurse, these practical lab classes are invaluable. It is where you learn the basics and also where you get the background for your work. You learn to give medications, proper injection techniques, how to implement proper hygiene, how to give first aid, and basically anything that you need to know that will allow you to care for the patient. The practice lab helps you get prepared to go to the hospital to work on real people.

DOING WELL IN CLINICAL LAB

For the first years, you will probably be subjected to classes where you are oriented about some of the most basic procedures that are used in Nursing. This will allow each student to expose themselves to the tasks that are entrusted to an actual Nurse.

Later on, actual hospital clinical labs are required. Students will do clinical labs in a hospital setting and the clinical instructors will be the ones to give the grades that are also equivalent to how you perform in an actual hospital work environment.

BUT HOW DO YOU DO WELL WITH SUCH A PRACTICAL APPROACH?

Well, you need to work towards a good work ethic. Don't make complaints all the time. Learn to get along with other nursing students and Nurses in the hospital.

Be open about the tasks that are given to you and give it your all. Utilize your critical thinking skills and be aware of time-management with your clinical skills. Don't do things halfheartedly and always follow the proper steps and hospital protocol. Your instructors will definitely take note of how you handle yourself in the workplace, so you should be aware of how to act and carry yourself. Be professional in the clinical setting and maintain patient confidentiality.

Doing well is not about getting the highest grades; rather, it's about the actual experience that you get to receive in this environment.

PROFESSIONAL NURSE SPOTLIGHT
THE CLINICAL EXPERIENCE

Nursing programs are primarily comprised of phases and components. Many schools have the pre-requisite phase and the clinical phase. In some programs, the students are required to take general education courses and required introductory courses or pre-requisite courses. Other schools have programs that start off with co-requisite courses where the students take nursing courses starting in the very first semester and proceed throughout the curriculum. In the curriculum I will discuss, there are two components. The students have a pre-requisite phase and a clinical phase. The clinical phase is comprised of three components: the lecture, the skills laboratory, and the clinical experience. The skills laboratory and the clinical experience components are the areas in which the students learn, practice, and demonstrate the psychomotor skills of Nursing.

The clinical experience occurs in a health care facility such as a hospital, nursing home, behavior health center, outpatient area, or a community facility. Students are exposed to patients at various stages of the wellness-illness continuum such as acute illness, long-term (chronic illness), mental health concerns, and wellness. Students also are exposed to patients in different developmental stages across the lifespan. Using Erick Ericson developmental stages which range from infancy to old age, the clinical experience introduces the student to each phase of development as they work with patients in various age groups.

The clinical experience allows the student to work with real live patients under the auspices of the clinical instructor.

The clinical instructor is an experienced Registered Nurse prepared at the master's degree or higher. The clinical instructor is affiliated with the School of Nursing and is completely aware of the nursing curriculum and what the student is required to learn. The clinical experience is aligned with the didactic and skills laboratory portions of the program.

The students will be provided with cognitive information in the didactic setting, demonstrate and practice the related psychomotor skill in the skills laboratory, and perform the skill under supervision in the clinical experience. To perform in the clinical experience, there are requirements of each student. There is an expectation that the student will practice the skill to be demonstrated prior to arriving at the clinical arena. The skills lab is set up with mannequins that the students will practice on and there are skills that the students can practice on each other. The student should not be practicing the skill for the first time in the healthcare facility. The clinical assignment should closely align with the skills in the lecture and skills lab for the week. The requirements to enter the clinical experience include pre-clinical preparation where the student is expected to look-up information on the patient's diagnoses and be prepared to discuss it in the pre-clinical conference.

The diagnoses are discussed in general terms with knowledge of what it is, how to take care of it, and the expected treatment that can be provided. The student must be prepared upon arrival at the clinical site.

Other requirements include being awake, astute, and aware of the patient and his/her needs. The student will need to be aware of the patient's medications and treatments, the stage of development, co-morbidity, and actual and potential nursing diagnosis. The student must come to the clinical area prepared with all homework assignments completed, dressed in appropriated attire or uniform, be on time, and with a desire to learn and excel. Basic to the uniform requirements are the attire approved by your nursing program which includes approved footwear, name tag, stethoscope and other required equipment, black pen, pocket note pad, clinical experience pocket guide which complements the textbook, a watch with a second hand and seconds marked off and the greatest desire to learn.

Nursing students should possess a positive attitude and a strong desire to learn while serving others. They should expect nothing in return other than the reward of successfully completing the nursing program and passing the NCLEX exam.

Frances E. Montague, APRN, MSN, RN-C Nursing Faculty, Virginia State University
Member -Virginia Nurse Association & Central VA Chapter - Black Nurses Association

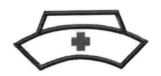

CHAPTER 17:
TEST SUCCESS

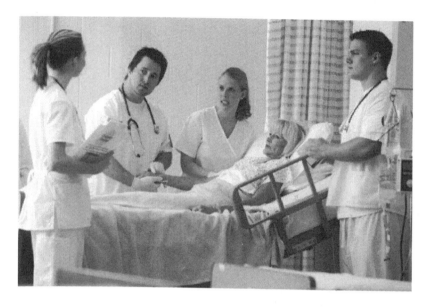

"Nurses don't wait until October to celebrate make a difference day –
They make a difference everyday" – Anonymous

A lot of people are always wondering about how nursing students actually get things right. With all those procedures, it's a wonder how the students are actually able to absorb them. But of course, not everyone is able to perfect it the first time. There will always be mistakes that will set you back a few paces, but the important thing is that you are able to evaluate the wrong that you did so you can correct it the next time.

MEASURING TEST SUCCESS IN LECTURE

Test success in lecture will depend on whether or not you are able to pass the testes or quizzes. Normally, students are given a test or quiz each week to evaluate if they are able to utilize the critical thinking skills of a Nurse.

Most Nursing Schools require the student to make an 80% on each test to be considered a passing grade. The student will be given a series of questions with multiple-choice answers. Critical thinking on the part of the student will become easier overtime and with practice.

Think like a Nurse to become a professional Nurse. What makes the thinking of a Nurse to think differently than, any other professions? As a Nurse you, will have to view the client/patient and their symptoms as a whole. Then, you are required to use what you have learned from your Nursing coursework; the ideas, concepts and theories of Nursing and related skills so that we become self-directed, critical thinkers to solve or prevent the patient's problems.

MEASURING TEST SUCCESS IN PRACTICE LAB

Let's say that you are required to work with partners to take a blood sample. How do you measure the test success for that? This will probably involve both of your inputs. You will be given instructions on how to perform it, the basics on why it is done, and to review the benefits.

The test success rate will depend on how you were able to perform it with the partner.

Did it hurt him?

Were you able to take just the right amount?

It's precision and skill together when you want to measure the success of a certain test. Your instructors will ask about how you did it and if you encountered any problems while performing the procedure. Don't be intimidated – speak your mind and talk to them clearly.

If you did something wrong, ask them about it. Maybe you applied the tourniquet too tight and that's why it hurt. Maybe you didn't follow proper protocol and your partner ended using the wrong blood tubes. These are common mistakes and everyone makes them.

Ask what went wrong and remedy it. The pass rate for every procedure that you do will only go up if you are able to perform it without any mistake the next time.

CHAPTER 18:
PERSONAL LIFE DURING
NURSING SCHOOL

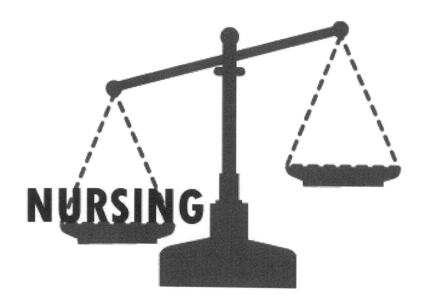

"I attribute my success to this:
I never gave or took any excuse" – Florence Nightingale

The personal life of a student nurse might not be as interesting as that of an art student, but there is definitely something to be said about their capability to balance all the aspects that come with school and other outside relationships.

SOCIAL

When it comes to friendly outings and get together events, nursing students might not be able to attend as much of these anymore.

The first years of school maybe, but as they progress further in school, these kinds of events will be less of a priority.

RELATIONSHIPS

So what happens to your love life then? This might be another compromise that you have to live with. Unless you already have your partner who is willing and understanding enough to consider your busy schedule, it will be quite hard to find a potential mate during this time. It will be a hectic two to four years and you have to set your eyes on the goal of graduating first.

STUDIES

This aspect will definitely become personal in your life in the next four years of Nursing School. Your lessons and academics are very important so in order to be good at what you do; you will need to prioritize this.

The reason why you won't be able to attend too much to your social and love relationships is because of this. It's part of the compromise that comes with being a nursing student.

PERSONAL TIME

This time will be limited while in Nursing School. Please have a schedule of fun activities that can be incorporated to promote relaxation. Even nursing students need to have a little fun, once in a while.

SPIRITUAL TIME IN YOUR PERSONAL AND PROFESSIONAL LIFE

Utilize your spiritual foundation, while in Nursing School. Continue to connect daily, before every test and before clinical with the Higher Power. During times of difficulty seek comfort with a Higher Power in your personal and professional life while in Nursing School and beyond.

PROFESSIONAL NURSE SPOTLIGHT
PERSONAL LIFE DURING NURSING SCHOOL

Whether it's curling up with a good book, cooking dinner with friends, or taking a regular yoga class, making time for a personal life and participating in self-care activities is vital to replenishing the nursing student's soul.

I remember those long days and late nights, meeting in study groups, reviewing everything from nursing theory and pathophysiology to pharmacology and therapeutic communication in mental health. Then, I'd have to go home exhausted from a long day of studying only to wake up and do it all over again. It seemed that there was so little time for anything else.

But, just like scheduling your study groups and adhering to your classroom schedule, it's also important to schedule out time for your personal life and self-care.

Here's a tip...

Schedule at least one group activity + one self-care activity per week.

Try scheduling these two activities on your days off from studying... and yes, days off are allowed! Scheduling these activities will also help improve your time management skills as well.

Participating in activities you love, whether it's for fun in groups or spending time alone, replenishes your mental and physical health, thus relieving stress and having you ready to take on your school- related tasks with greater ease.

Also, participating in group activities that are non-nursing related, gives you the opportunity to connect with your peers in healthy, non-stressful ways.

Here are some activities you can try:

- Yoga

- Meditation

- Hiking

- a Book Club

- Ultimate Frisbee

- Music Lessons

- Reiki Therapy

Another tip…

It's okay to say 'No.'

As much as human connection is important for overall well-being, having boundaries in place can also keep you sane when you're truly limited on time and energy.

When you're asked to devote your time or energy to other people or projects during your free time, remember it's okay to decline…

no matter what they may think of you. Saying 'no' to requests that you don't have the extra time for or even want to do is about taking care of yourself. And those who care about you will understand your need to take a time-out when you just need a break.

So make a commitment to yourself; take care of you!

Marsha Battee, RN is a Lifestyle Design Strategist who is passionate about helping nurses start their own businesses. As the founder of, "The Bossy Nurse," Marsha blogs on business strategies, insight and inspiration to help Nurses live a life full of happiness, health and freedom. She also owns and operates her own boutique travel company where Nurses "travel for fun…not work" at www. RNgetaways.com.

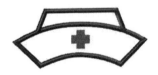

CHAPTER 19:
KEYS TO NURSING
SUCCESS

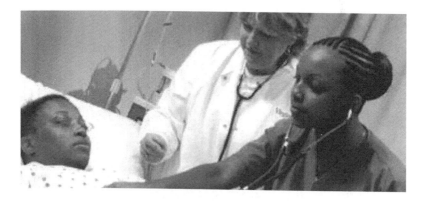

*"They may forget your name, but will
never forget the way you made them feel."*
- Maya Angelo

So a lot of students and potential students are probably thinking about what really makes for a successful run in Nursing School. After all, Nursing is no easy course to tackle. In a span of a few years, you will have to master all the basics so that you are prepared to face the professional world after graduation. Let's talk about some basic factors that can influence your success, both in Nursing School and in your career afterwards.

BELIEF

Nothing is worse than a Nurse who is driven by panic – leave this to the patients. As early as the first years in Nursing School, train yourself to become ready for anything. Whether it's that unexpected quiz or an emergency situation in a hospital, how you carry yourself will be a determining factor in the results. Don't let yourself be run by emotions. Be calm and alert so that you are still able to function and be productive in spite of many unexpected circumstances that may come your way. Believe it and you can achieve it!

CONFIDENCE

Whether you are still a nursing student or already a professional, one thing that you have to take heart is the motivation to never stop learning. Despite the two to four years in school that will be used up for this purpose, the journey to being a Nurse does not end there. There are so many more concepts and other specialties that you can take up afterwards. It is one of the advantages of entering a career path that is both broad and versatile.

Just because you have your license and you are already working, it doesn't mean that you have to stay there forever. Learn about new methods and some concepts that can help you out so that you can grow and have more room for improvement. Be confident, you can do this!!

SELF-DISCIPLINE

There is no doubt that Nursing will be one of the harder courses that you will ever encounter in school. It is a mix of both theory and practical application after all. And in order to succeed, you need a good idea of what self-discipline is and how to implement it in your life. This will be your greatest weapon against a bombardment of tasks. With self-discipline, you will be able to classify each task according to your priority so that you will not have any delays. Maintain self-discipline to be successful.

SELF-KNOWLEDGE

Never be a closed-minded person when you intend to become a Nurse. By doing this, you will also be closing yourself off to many opportunities. As you progress through Nursing School, there are times when instructors teach by unconventional means, but this does not mean that you can condemn them; rather, it's a prompt that you have to learn to adapt. In the nursing profession, you will be faced with a lot of hard decisions. In order to cope, you need to open up to new policies or changes so that you will not end up at an impasse. It's important to be flexible! Use your self-knowledge to get through.

PROFESSIONAL NURSE SPOTLIGHT
KEYS TO NURSING SUCCESS

"It is natural for youth to be full of hope and full of confidence, and to think that the present is more important than the past, and it is natural for young nurses to think their elders who advise are croakers and wet blankets." 1 This observation, expressed by a nurse in 1935, shows that generational differences in Nursing are far from new.

I suggest that there are three keys to your Nursing success, and they are the multigenerational workforce, strategic partnering, and resilience. Let's visit them individually.

The first key to your Nursing success is learning how to cope in a multigenerational work setting and to be a voice for Nurses and Nursing. Communication styles and work preferences of Nurses vary consistently with their generation, education, and upbringing. Your key is to know how to work with those who prefer face- to-face discussions and staff meetings, and with those who prefer email and texting. Think about how you and your colleagues like to give and receive feedback.

For example, the boomers are independent, critical thinkers with a strong work ethic. The millennials in your workplace like to work in teams, but also crave instant rewards, recognition and more. Learn how to engage with these professionals and to keep them motivated. Realize and appreciate the differences and how this information will impact patient care, outcomes, and productivity in your nursing workplace.

Stimson, the author of the 1935 article, was a connector for Nurses. In Malcolm Gladwell's book, The Tipping Point, he addresses those with vast networks of people in various personal and professional pools who hear new ideas, talk about them, and share them, as connectors. Within Nursing, we have many examples of tipping points. The Magnet hospital movement, the advanced nurse practitioner, and nursing specialization are all tipping points. As a new Nurse, think about the tipping points of which you are aware and how they will influence the choices that you make in your career. Many of the 'connectors' with large networks will possibly become your strategic partners.

Strategic partnering, within and beyond institutions, provides opportunities for personal and professional growth, outreach, and collaboration. That is what we, as Nurses, do...and we do it well! Leaders, such as yourselves, hear new ideas, talk about them, and share them with your counterparts. Your counterparts around the country and across the globe have challenged the process, forged strategic partnerships with their nursing peers, and created excellence. They are resilient.

Resilience is a skill that can be learned. It will empower you to bounce back after providing care to others, after long study periods, after long shifts. Resilience is your ability to adjust to adversity, to build strong professional relationships, achieve work/life balance, and improve your work environment. Workplace adversity is often associated with lack of autonomy, bullying, organizational issues, nursing shortages and more.

As a Nurse, you will be with clients and their families through all phases of life. As the healthcare system continues to change, and as the settings in which care is provided expand, personal resilience will enhance your ability to cope.

To thrive and survive in such an environment, we must be resilient. Resilience is the third key to your nursing success. Use it wisely!

Consider the three keys and use them to refine your understanding of Nursing; allow them to help you as you explore the exceptional opportunities available to you as a nursing professional. You are the future…you are your own success!

Enjoy a day of abundance and share the gift of health and wealth with those whose lives you impact!

Sharon M. Weinstein, MS, RN, CRNI, FACW, FAAN Founder of SMW Group LLC Integrative Health Forum

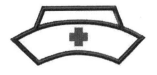

CHAPTER 20:
CULTURE IN NURSING SCHOOL

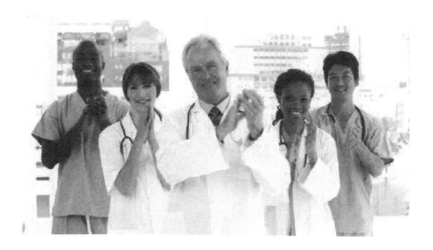

"It would not be possible to praise a nurse too highly"
– Stephen Ambrose

As early as Nursing School, a student is already taught about the culture of being a Nurse. No matter what school you attend, there is one principle that will be taught and enforced strictly: SAFETY FIRST.

Doing practice lab and clinical in hospitals is a part of the curriculum of most Nursing Schools. This allows their students to train for the real thing. They will be under the supervision of

Professional Nurses during this time and they are taught about how things are in a real work environment.

For these students, it is ingrained in them that the patients they are dealing with are real people. They cannot just make assumptions about the diagnosis or go ahead and proceed without following protocol as this can lead to conflicts and troubles. Any miscalculation can be detrimental to the patient that they are taking care of. Safety is an utmost priority in the hospital. Even in Nursing School, this has already grown to be a part of its culture, aside from the academic curriculum.

CULTURE IN NURSING SCHOOL FOR NURSING STUDENTS THAT MUST BE MAINTAINED:

- Address instructors with respect and by last name

- Maintain the school uniform and dress code

- Refrain from inappropriate social media dialog

- Adhere to confidentiality policies

- Avoid illegal activities

- Remember SAFETY FIRST!

PHASE 3:
INTERVIEW WITH NURSING STUDENTS

The key to success for any nursing student is like two sides of a coin – it will depend on how the person handles the affairs and requirements that are needed to pass every subject. Let us further explore the in-depth reasons as to what really makes a successful and an unsuccessful nursing student.

CHAPTER 21:
SUCCESSFUL NURSING
STUDENTS

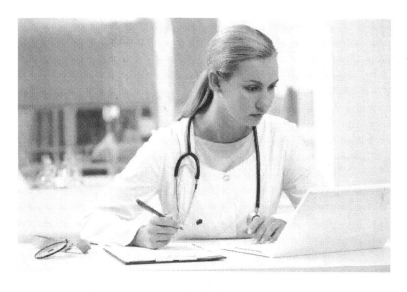

"No matter how difficult the days may get,
never forget the reason you became a nurse" – Anonymous

Achieving success and recognition as a student nurse is not easily done by achieving high grades. You need to be a wholesome package for both academics and practical procedures. It's a balance of both that will propel you to succeed. Here are some good traits of that can help you understand what it really means to be a successful nursing student.

A GOOD OUTLOOK

One of the best traits to possess in Nursing School is a positive attitude. Giving off good vibes also allows for more positive feelings to flow within you. Even if you are tired, you will continue to be productive in more ways than one because of this good outlook in life.

A Nurse is tough. Although they may be weary from all the work and caring for patients, they continue to do their job with precision and grace. This positive perspective does wonders for both students and professionals.

A DREAMER

Setting your sight on the goal is the best way to succeed in Nursing. Do you want to be a Registered Nurse? Then work for it. Be a dreamer and work your way up to the top. Think of Nursing School as a ladder that will bring you to the top of your career.

A HARD WORKER

As they say, hardworking people can beat even the smartest ones. In a course like Nursing, no matter how good you are at memorizing concepts, you have to understand that there are still practical procedures to consider. Working hard to balance both aspects is very important if you want to succeed in the course over the next few years.

NURSING STUDENT INTERVIEW ON SUCCESS

I met with a group of recent graduates for lunch. Some have passed all their classes the first time and some had to repeat a class before they were able to graduate. Everyone agreed that Nursing School is hard work, but they loved it. Thanks for meeting with me!!

Question # 1

What helped you succeed in Nursing School?

Dana L. – "Never slack off in Nursing School. The same dedication it took to get into Nursing School is the same dedication it will take to pass each class and complete Nursing School."

Dee. M. – "I have a passion for Nursing and feel, it is my calling."

Question # 2

What tips would you give others to help pass a test?

Michelle R. – "Put in the time to study and stay organized with your notes."

Wanda G. – "Do not go out and party, the night before a test."

Question # 3

What would you tell someone who is interested in Nursing School?

Donna B. – "This is the biggest sacrifice of your life."

Daniel K. – "Find a nursing mentor, before you start the clinical phase."

Question # 4

Do successful nursing students have a social life?

Dana L. – "Truthfully No! To pass, you have to stick to a schedule and limit your non-nursing activities. Eat, sleep and then Nursing School is the norm."

Dee M. – "No, I did not have the time. I am hoping to start dating, after I pass the NCLEX. Maybe I will meet someone at work."

Question #5

Do successful nursing students work while in school?

Michelle R. – "Yes, I worked as a Nurse Tech only one day every other week."

Wanda G. – "No, I tried that last time and it was too much for me."

Question # 6

What would you have done differently to pass Nursing School easier?

Donna B. – "I would have the syllabus and books before school started and make a study plan early for the entire semester."

Daniel K. – "I would have educated my family on the limited time I had outside of school."

CHAPTER 22: UNSUCCESSFUL NURSING STUDENTS

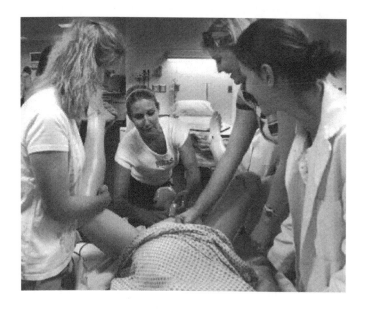

"We'd all be worse without a nurse "– Anonymous

So what makes an unsuccessful student nurse? Here are some signs that you should watch out for and avoid:

A PROCRASTINATOR

Another no-no for nursing students is procrastination. Are you putting away your tasks for today just because you have time tomorrow? Think again.

Any student who is taking up nursing will not have such luxury. You might be able to put off some of your work today, but it will get back to you tenfold. By the next day, you will have another batch of tasks to finish and make up for another round of duty hours. You will end up severely behind because you will be stuck doing the tasks of yesterday instead of being an efficient worker.

Cramming is not a good attitude to have in nursing. Lagging behind in lessons and practical applications will affect your productivity and this is simply not an option if you wish to pass the course without any troubles.

A FAULTFINDER

Another trait of an unsuccessful nursing student is being a faultfinder. Basically, this person is the one who is always complaining. "I'm tired", "This is so hard", "I can't do this" are only some of the most common statements that you hear from these people.

For every task that they are assigned to do, they always find fault. Perhaps it's their way of coping with the difficulties of the course or maybe they are just not committed enough. Either way, this negative attitude will eventually erode their way to success.

For obvious reasons, nursing students that are like this will probably end up failing. But then again, they will also find excuses for that too!

A "YES" PERSON

Many of you may wonder how this has been categorized as negative when saying yes seems to give a good impression.

Well, when you are a nursing student, things are a bit different. Duties will be passed on to you and together with lessons and social obligations on the side, some students simply cannot afford to say yes to more tasks.

If your friends are asking you to go out or there is some event that you need to go to, say no if it will end up affecting your schedule. If someone is asking you to help him or her with lessons, say no if you yourself are also behind. Don't be afraid to voice your opinion and stand your ground.

Prioritizing is the key to success in nursing. You have to know which tasks are the most important ones and which ones you can set aside for the next time.

NURSING STUDENT INTERVIEW
ON UNSUCCESS

I met with a group of recent graduates for lunch. Some had passed all their classes the first time and some had to repeat a class before they were able to graduate. Everyone agreed that Nursing School is hard work, but they loved it.

Question # 1
Why were you unsuccessful in a class in Nursing School?

Dana L. – "I did not ask for help, when I failed the first test." Dee. M. – "I did not want to change the way I normally studied

for classes."

Question # 2
What did you see students do, who were unsuccessful in

Nursing School?

Michelle R. – "They were late to class and do not take notes in class."

Wanda G. – "They were late to clinical and did not complete clinical prep."

Question # 3
What would you tell someone who is afraid of failing Nursing

School?

Donna B. – "Know your weakness and strengths in school up front."

Daniel K. – "Have a strong foundation in the basic science and anatomy classes."

Question # 4
What was positive about failing a nursing class?

Dana L. – "It made me try harder to succeed the second time around."

Dee. M. – "I realized I had to change to become a Nurse."

PHASE 4: GRADUATION & PASSING THE NCLEX

Is it the end of the road for you now that graduation is looming in the horizon? There are so many things that come into mind when you think about graduation after four years of studying. But for Nurses, this phase is not yet done. In fact, it might be another chapter of learning for them since they have to review for the upcoming licensure exams.

The NCLEX is the universal requirement for all Nurses. It is the licensure exam that will provide you with the title of Registered Nurse (RN). It will be the proof that you are qualified to work with real people. Before you can work as a Nurse, you will need to pass this exam first. Let us explore this line of thought further in the next chapters.

CHAPTER 23:
GRADUATION PLAN/
ENJOY

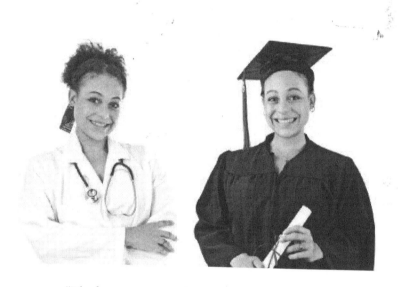

*"The best nurses are those that go the extra mile,
even when no one is on the sidelines watching"*
– Anonymous

Graduation and receiving that diploma is probably the highest point for every nursing student. After all the struggles that you might have experienced during the past four years, this is only natural. But graduation is not merely another chapter that ends. It is also another beginning.

You will now be carving your path into becoming a Professional Nurse.

Do enjoy some break time after you have graduated, but after that, decide and plan out the next steps in your career. It's another rocky path that you have to undergo because similar to Nursing School, uncertainties will surely be there.

You will have to study again and pass the NCLEX.

NURSING STUDENT INTERVIEW ON GRADUATION

I met with a group of recent graduates over lunch. Everyone agreed that Nursing School is hard work, but they loved it. They were still excited about the graduation.

Question # 1
What was it like to graduate from Nursing School?

Dana L. – "It was an amazing experience to receive my nursing pin."

Dee. M. – "I shed tears of joy for myself and my classmates. It was beautiful"

Question # 2
Who did you dedicate your nursing school success to?

Michelle R. – "My parents! I received a lot of financial help from them."

Wanda G. – "My babysitter! She watched my kids for me all the time."

Question # 3

What did you like best about the pinning ceremony?

Donna B. – "I liked the songs that we requested during the ceremony."

Daniel K. – "I enjoyed the speaker. She was very inspirational."

CHAPTER 24:
PLANNING & PASSING
THE NCLEX

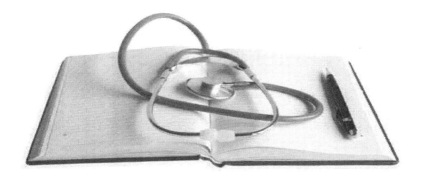

"Nursing is not a job; it's an adventure" – Anonymous

WHAT HAPPENS AFTER GRADUATION FOR NURSING STUDENTS?

THE NCLEX HAPPENS NEXT.

This is the licensure exam that every aspiring Nurse needs to pass before they are allowed to work in hospitals and medical clinics. Unlike other careers, those who do not get a license will also lose the opportunity to be called a Registered Nurse.

SO WHAT DOES NCLEX ENTAIL? HOW DO YOU START STUDYING?

The first thing that you need to do is decide whether you are going to review solo or take classes for it. There are some review centers that you can enroll in to help you out with the basic concepts.

If you are not sure about which route to take, ask some people you know. Approach and ask your mentors and other RNs in your area about their experiences prior to the NCLEX so that you can get an idea of what to expect. This will constitute that whole planning stage before the exam.

HOW DO I PASS THE NCLEX?

There is no foolproof method for anyone. You'll have to work hard for it. Diligence is the key. All your lessons from your first year to the last will have to be reviewed and understood thoroughly if you want that chance at passing and becoming a Registered Nurse.

Read books and listen to lectures. Study how the test is supposed to be given and try out some mock tests beforehand to know your aptitude on several subjects. Find out where you are weak and work on that area.

Always remember to PRAY!!!

NURSING STUDENT INTERVIEW ON PASSING NCLEX

I met with a group of recent graduates over lunch. Everyone agreed that Nursing School is hard work, but they loved it. They were still excited about passing the NCLEX.

Question # 1
What was the NCLEX like?

Dana L. – "I was so scared to take that test."

Dee. M. – "I was nervous and glad to learn I pass the test."

Question # 2
How did you prepare to take the NCLEX?

Michelle R. – "I took the suggested review from the school, we graduated from."

Wanda G. – "I kept a study schedule, to pass the NCLEX."

Question # 3
What would you tell someone who's getting ready to take the NCLEX?

Donna B. – "Do what you did to pass the other tests in Nursing School."

Daniel K. – "Eat breakfast, pray and be on time for the NCLEX test."

CHAPTER 25:
STUDY HABITS AND TIME MANAGEMENT

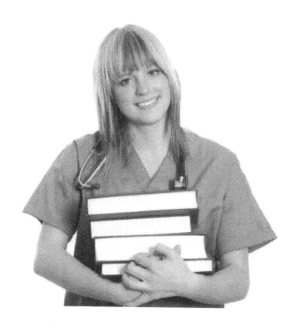

"You never know who needs you. Good energy is contagious" -
Anonymous

Remember those late-night cramming sessions you had during school? Unfortunately, they do not end here. After you receive your diploma, you will need to work on passing the test for your license to become a Professional Nurse.

The NCLEX, as your next step, will probably require a collective effort on your part to squeeze out all that stored knowledge that you were able to absorb in the past years.

This licensure exam will "test" your practice. Without it, you won't be able to work as a professional nurse, so it goes without saying that you should put that best foot forward.

Alleviate all the unnecessary distractions that will cause you to lose your focus. Set specific times for your study hours and adhere to a strict schedule. During your short time of reviewing, it is imperative that you spend it learning some things over and over again.

Together with good study habits, you will also need to incorporate effective time management. They go hand in hand in helping you keep up with all the lessons that you need to review. Setting priorities will be the biggest factor in helping you study.

When you are already in the NCLEX stage, it is necessary to change your study habits. You have to be more vigilant and focused on what needs to be done because most teachers in review centers will not be spoon-feeding you. They will serve as guides, but you are basically on your own on this endeavor.

PROFESSIONAL NURSE SPOTLIGHT
GRADUATION AND PASSING THE NCLEX

Whenever you hear an instructor say, "This is something you need to know for the NCLEX," write it down. Write it in a separate notebook and save these tidbits of information for your review time. This will be a valuable piece of your study guide for the NCLEX.

One of the things I always recommend to students is to establish a group of study buddies during your clinical rotations. And before you graduate, set up a schedule to review together for the NCLEX. Have each person take a topic and prepare a review lesson for the group. Use the popular study guides available such as Mosby's, Kaplan's, etc., and make flash cards, design a practice test and go over the right and wrong answers as a group. Take a practice online test together and discuss the answers. Keep it casual and NON-JUGEMENTAL. Support each other and offer a different way to consider or remember things. Everyone learns in a different way and perhaps one of your peers can help you understand something the best of teachers failed to get across.

By Kathy Quan RM BSN PHN
Founder of TheNursingSite.com and TheNursingSiteBlog.com
Author: The Everything New Nurse Book, The New Nurse Handbook &150 Tips and Tricks for New Nurses

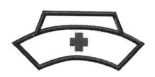

PHASE 5: THE "NOVICE TO EXPERT" NURSE

WHAT MAKES AN EXPERT NURSE?

This part of the book will talk about the most important factor that is involved from the evolution of being a novice to becoming an expert.

There are so many nursing school grads that pass the NCLEX and think they are ready to practice as a Nurse. You will be so scared on your first job. In the beginning, you are a "Novice Nurse". Everything is new. It takes time to become an "Expert Nurse".

CHAPTER 26:
NOVICE TO EXPERT
NURSE

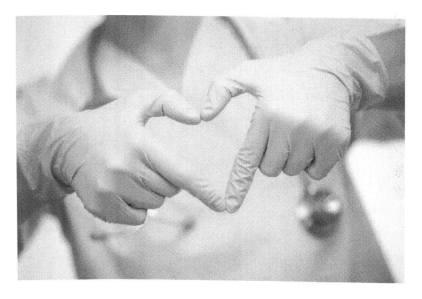

"I am thankful to be a nurse because I can touch someone's life in a moment and create a lasting impression" – Unknown

What is the difference between the "novice and the expert"? It all comes down to one thing: EXPERIENCE!

The more cases that you are able to handle over a period of time, the more knowledge you gain about what to do in various situations.

As a nursing student, you will be required to assist the professionals in the hospital, and you will slowly be exposed to a wide selection of diagnosis for different patients.

Although theories and lessons give you a good background about what Nursing is all about, nothing is as good as practical application. When you see the symptoms for yourself, you can make better deductions.

The same is true for emergencies. It's normal for "novice" Nurses to have the tendency to panic. But those who have been a Nurse for a long time know that resorting to such emotions will only cause unproductive results. You have been trained to become more resilient in times of adversity.

Expose yourself to different environments and do not be afraid to go out of your comfort zone. Take time to learn even if it is tough. Learning from books can only give you so much information; but when you acquire practical know-hows, you gain so much more in terms of experience.

Aside from certifications and taking some licensure exams, the only way that you can really become an "expert nurse" is to build up on time and experience.

Why do you think those "older" Nurses come off as a very soothing presence in front of their patients?

PROFESSIONAL NURSE SPOTLIGHT
"NOVICE TO EXPERT" NURSE

Whenever we think about Nurses, we often think about a "licensed" Nurse who "knows the drill" and "knows exactly what to do" in any given situation.

Believe it or not, becoming a fully functional Nurse is a process – it takes many hours of working in real-life situations to develop that expertise. It's normal and natural for all new nursing students (even new Nurses) to feel a bit of anxiety when they first perform a skill, meet a patient, or make a nursing decision. What's important to remember is that every Nurse was once a "newbie".

When I think about my own career as a Nurse, I can vividly remember my first day of Nursing School, as well as my first day on my first nursing job, even my first time teaching a Nursing Lecture to nursing students. My how I've changed throughout the years!

Some experts argue that it takes up to 10 years of full-time work to become an expert. I think that it takes a humble-minded person full of confidence to eventually develop in to a full-fledged expert. If one has the ability to learn new things, add to their "toolbox" over time, and learn from others more experienced than themselves, they can continually develop their own skills and abilities.

In Nursing, even experienced Nurses find themselves as a "newbie" once again when they start a new job in a new area, pursue a new path in Nursing, or return to school.

In Nursing, we learn new things each and every day. It's what makes Nursing a great career choice.

What's around your next bend in the road? If you remain committed and stay the course, you'll find amazing things ahead!

Amber McCall, PhD, FNP-BC, RN Assistant Professor
Georgia Regents University

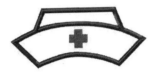

PHASE 6:
THE FUTURE OF NURSING

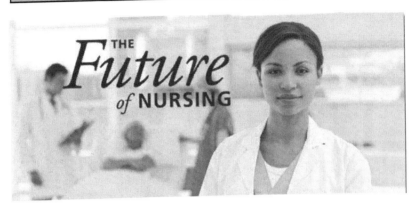

"I am thankful to be a nurse because I get to advocate for people who are at their weakest" – Heidi R.

What happens when you have that job as a Registered Nurse? Is that the end line for you? Don't be pessimistic. There are still so many opportunities that can come your way even if you are done with getting that Bachelor's Degree.

Be open-minded and try to seek out other options and career routes that you can take as a Professional Nurse. It's a whole new struggle that you have to go through so that you can make your way up to the top.

Contrary to popular belief, Nurses are not merely limited to work in the hospital. There are a variety of fields that you can get into after passing the licensure exam. This part will help you sift through the possibilities when it comes to furthering your career and earning big as a Nurse.

CHAPTER 27:
CAREERS IN NURSING

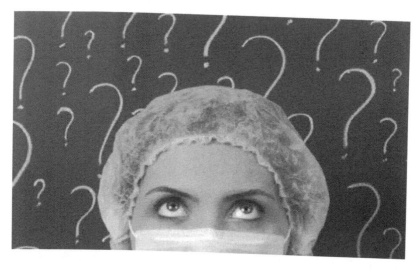

"Nurses are the hospitality of the hospital" – Carrie Late

Nursing is a broad career path. Upon graduation and acquiring your license, you will be presented with a variety of choices and positions that you can hold as a Registered Nurse. You may decide to work in a hospital or a clinic, while others may decide to become Private Nurses. It's a matter of choosing the right position where you are most comfortable.

Here are some possible positions that can be obtained by Registered

Nurses:

- Midwife

- Clinical Nurse

- Anesthetist

- Educator

- Practitioner

- Staff Nurse

There are also different types of nursing specialties that you can go for. Much like how Doctors can be diverse in their chosen specialty, Nurses also have this option. You can get various certifications and training courses that will help you get the title of a "specialized" Nurse. This will widen your scope or practice and allow you to work in different sectors aside from the hospital.

As a career, getting a specialization will also open more doors to success. Only a few people go for these options and when you are a rarity, you will be in demand.

Here is a list of some of the nursing specialties that you can take up:

- AIDS Care

- Infection Specialist and Control

- Neuroscience

- Occupational Therapy

- Oncology

- Ophthalmology

- Orthopedics

- Pediatrics

- Psychiatric Nurse

- Reconstructive Surgery

- Rehabilitation

- School Nurse

- Renal

GOING FOR ALTERNATIVES

Now, if you are interested in a more unconventional route for your career as a Nurse, you might want to consider some alternative choices. These are not the typical choice that most people make, but they do make for a more interesting alternative than the usual nursing job.

You can be a Flight Nurse, a Military Nurse, a Forensic Nurse, or a Travel Nurse. You will most likely be required to stay on duty for longer hours, but if you are after practical experience, these are good choices because you will be exposed to a wider variety of situations.

Straying even farther away, you can even make a living as a nurse/health consultant or a nurse/health writer. Nursing school, your qualifications and license will give you the credibility you need to jumpstart your career in these other sectors, thus affording you a lot of opportunities to hone your skills.

All in all, you have really nothing to fear if you can't get a job in a local hospital. Most people think that just because there are Nurses that can't get jobs, then it makes for a hopeless situation; but this is not true. You can make your own career path as a professional Nurse and there are definitely so many industries that you can enter.

If you do not like to be placed in hectic duties in a hospital, then it might be more feasible to look for other workplaces. Go for clinics or seek out other alternatives. Don't be afraid to explore. From being a specialist to setting up your own special care clinic, it's just a matter of knowing more and choosing a job that you will love for the years to come. There are plenty of careers in Nursing to choose from.

PROFESSIONAL NURSE SPOTLIGHT
CAREERS IN NURSING

Since my early years in elementary school, I had a desire to pursue a career in Nursing. I believe that nursing is a "calling" or a "gift" that I share with others. I started my journey 19 years ago as a Licensed Practical Nurse and then transitioned to become a professional Registered Nurse. Nursing is not just a job but also a career that you can hold near and dear to your heart for life. Today, I am currently Masters prepared in Nursing and Health Care Informatics. I am also Certified in Acute Care Case Management and served in the Army Reserves as a Nurse Officer for 4 years. Informatics is a field that is growing for Nurses because of the growth of technology, the trend to decrease healthcare cost, and increase quality and outcomes. I always had a love for computers and technology. Informatics has given me an avenue to bring nursing experience, leadership experience, and technology full circle making this career move very satisfying.

What is Nursing Informatics? Nursing Informatics is a specialty that integrates nursing science, computer science, and information science to manage and communicate data, information, knowledge, and wisdom in nursing practice (Nursing Informatics: Scope and Standards of Practice, ANA 2008). We support consumers, patients, nurses, healthcare providers, and other roles in the decision making process for inclusion of data sources in the electronic health record or information technology system. This career will need Nurses to have a pretty detailed background in

Nursing before pursuing this path. Most employers will require at the minimum a Bachelor's Degree in Nursing or Informatics. However, there are occasions that employers will accept an Associate's Degree in Nursing. Nurse

Informaticists play a crucial role in developing, implementing, and optimizing clinical application systems for electronic health records. According to the 2014 survey of Nurse Informaticists, it suggests that we must have a solid background and experience to bring to their positions (HIMMS 2014 Nursing Informatics Workforce Survey). Training and education in Informatics continues to advance. Certification in Informatics is also available. Certification in any field demonstrates that you possess the credibility, marketability, and personal satisfaction in your field and shows that you value what you are doing which validates your specialized knowledge.

Nursing Informaticists job responsibilities may or may not have a supervisory role. Job roles can include computer system implementation and development, system utilization and optimization. Nursing Informatics can take you away from direct patient care but it helps you to focus on quality and safety of all patients. Personal skills needed for this position can include leadership skills, change management skills, knowledge of Governance structures within your organization, customer service skills, and knowledge of project management as well. As a Nurse, I feel satisfied in knowing that technology changes lives in many ways and we can leverage this technology to increase education about health and wellness and engage the consumer in their own care.

Andree Aboite, MSN-INF, RN
Clinical Informatics Specialists – VCU Health Systems
President, Central Virginia Chapter - Black Nurses Association

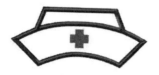

PROFESSIONAL NURSE SPOTLIGHT
CAREERS IN NURSING

Healthcare in general is constantly evolving and changing. New technology and the ever-constant need to cut costs dictate much of the change.

In recent years, Nurses have assumed more and more responsibility for patient education. Patients who understand their conditions and how they need to prevent complications will, in and of themselves, help to lower the costs of their own healthcare.

More than 50% of the population have no clue about healthcare and how to access it, how to prevent complications and promote wellness, nor what follow up they may need. This is healthcare illiteracy and it is a huge challenge for the nursing profession to solve.

It is said that the paradigm is shifting and that home healthcare will become what hospital nursing has been for almost 200 years. The majority of nursing careers will shift. Home Health Nursing is about making intermittent visits to patient's homes to observe them in their own environment and teach them how to care for themselves.

Whether it's diet and lifestyle changes or how to dress a wound and report any significant changes, this is an emerging trend. High tech tasks such as IV's, ventilator care, and pleurevacs are already part of the norm.

Patients are much sicker, yet many have been sent home or never qualified for hospital stays. These patients need professional help in order to learn how to care for themselves at home.

By Kathy Quan, RN BSN PHN
Founder: TheNursingSite.com and TheNursingSIteBlog.com
Author: The Everything New Nurse Book, The New Nurse Handbook & 150 Tips and Tricks for New Nurses

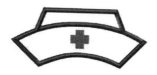

PROFESSIONAL NURSE SPOTLIGHT
CAREERS IN NURSING

The nursing profession is in a state of flux. With a rapidly aging population, healthcare reform, and seismic shifts in the world economy, Nurses must remain flexible, savvy, and fully aware of the forces shaping the profession---and the healthcare industry at large.

As hospitals downsize, close, or otherwise consolidate, Nurses are realizing that the traditional route of graduation from Nursing School followed by two years of med-surg is quickly becoming a notion from the past. While it's true that many employers and facilities have yet to read the "writing on the wall", the reality is that many new nursing graduates simply cannot manage to find med-surg positions with which to begin their careers.

In this shifting landscape, both Nurses and employers must both be flexible. In that regard, employers must provide the training and support that new Nurses need, especially those "novice" Nurses who are unable to launch their nursing careers with the previously coveted med-surg experience.

Meanwhile, Nurses must retool their expectations, approaching the job market with new eyes and a fresh perspective. This may involve doing more networking than they may have expected to do, or looking for more "non-traditional" first nursing positions, be it in corrections, primary care, home care, biotech, insurance nursing, occupational health, gerontology, forensics, or medical aesthetics.

Yes, the landscape is shifting under our feet, and the old paradigms simply no longer apply!

EXPANDING PRACTICE

With Advanced Practice Registered Nurses (APRNs) now having the ability to practice autonomously without physician oversight in more than 20 states, the scope of practice for Nurses has expanded exponentially.

With an increasing shortage of primary care physicians in many regions of the country, Nurse Practitioners are stepping in as primary providers for countless Americans, and anecdotal evidence demonstrates that NPs are viewed quite favorably by their patients.

Even Registered Nurses are realizing increased autonomy and a richer, more satisfying professional experience in a variety of settings. Thus, the world of nursing practice continues to expand.

NURSE ENTREPRENEURSHIP

In these early years of the 21st century, many Nurses are realizing that they can leverage their skills, relative autonomy, and professional credibility in order to venture into the world of Nurse Entrepreneurship.

Throughout the Unites States (and, presumably, other countries, as well) Nurses are launching businesses, including private practices as coaches and case managers, holistic practitioners, consultants, or owners of nursing agencies. Nurse entrepreneurs are developing and marketing products, working as professional writers or bloggers, or otherwise using their nursing skills and experience in ventures outside of traditional roles.

Training programs for fledgling Nurse Entrepreneurs have blossomed on the Internet, and there are business coaches who now realize that Nurses with an entrepreneurial spirit are excellent candidates for coaching and startup support services.

Nurse entrepreneurship will doubtless continue to grow in the decades to come, and an increasing number of Nurses will choose to either leave the bedside entirely upon entering the business world, or at least launch a satisfying side project that can supplement their nursing income.

SHIFTING PARADIGMS

In my own experience, I have chosen to continue to work part-time as a Registered Nurse while also pursuing various entrepreneurial projects.

My business ventures include working as a professional nurse writer, blogger and podcaster, as well as managing a practice as a Board Certified Nurse Coach who specifically provides career coaching for Nurses and healthcare professionals. I also serve as a speaker at nursing conferences, and I have a small consulting business in collaboration with another Nurse Entrepreneur.

The depth and breadth of what 21st century Nurses can achieve continues to expand and grow. With increased scopes of practice, entrepreneurial endeavors, and increasing opportunities to move beyond traditional nursing, there are literally no boundaries in terms of the employment outlook for Nurses.

The recognition that the old paradigms of nursing employment are crumbling is key. Meanwhile, flexibility, an open mind, and

the ability to read the "tea leaves" are essential for the Nurse who wishes to remain standing on the shifting ground upon which we find ourselves.

Stay aware, remain open, and embrace the new paradigms that the 21st century is offering to Nurses who "heed the call".

Keith Carlson, RN, BSN, NC-BC
Board Certified Nurse Coach, Nurse Blogger,
Podcaster and Speaker

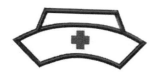

CHAPTER 28:
6-FIGURE CAREERS
IN NURSING

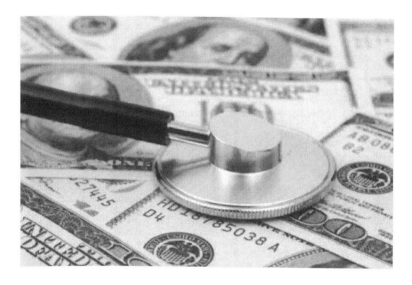

"Nursing: It's a beautiful thing when a career and a passion come together "- Anonymous

Some people have the impression that nursing is all about playing assistant to Doctors in a hospital. This is why most Nurses are not really held in high regard unless you have a high position in the workplace. But really, each one of those Nurses come with the right qualification; and with the right career choices, they can also earn six-figure salaries.

Did you think that only businessmen and athletes are capable of earning such big money?

WRONG!

Nurses too, can have superpowers in generating income. Much like how any career progresses, you'll have to work your way up to the top. There are so many career choices and routes that you can go for after getting your license, but if you really want to earn big, you'll have to step up your game as well.

Aside from getting a stable job, don't stop learning. Get more and more certifications as you can. Learn specialties. Get a Master's or Doctorate Degree, if you must. All of these will guarantee you better income in the future.

But once again, do not expect the road to success to be easy. Six-figure salaries are hard to achieve and it may take you as much as ten years to finally reach the peak of your career. As I said, you have to make your way to the top. It will not be instant gratification, that's for sure.

NURSING CAREER CHOICES WITH THE BIGGEST INCOME

So now, you have finally decided to work hard for that six-figure income and you probably want to know which among the many nursing specialties will help you achieve that. Advance Practice Nurses, Anesthetists, Clinical Nurse Specialists, and Midwives are four of the basic occupations that you can go for.

Take note though, there is no guarantee of earning big. It will also depend on how you handle your job and where you work.

Considering that most of these specialties require a lot of certifications and further learning, it can only be assumed that you'll have to work harder to be qualified for the title.

IS YOUR LOCATION SUITABLE?

There are some places that have a shortage with some specialty nurses, and this in turn, makes them a really valuable asset for both private practices and hospitals. This is one of the factors that can help you earn that six-figure income. You have to be particular about where you work so that you know what kind of Nurse is in demand.

SETTING UP YOUR OWN CLINIC

Another option that you can consider is to set up your own clinic. You may not be a medical doctor, but specialty nurses can also have their own clinics. As long as you are equipped with the right licenses, you can go for private practice.

One good example for this type of option is Midwifery. Most Certified Midwives do not really work in hospitals, but they have their own place where they can entertain patients all the same. Since there are still so many people who are quite averse with paying extra service fees that are charged in a hospital, you will have a lot of patients coming through if you choose to go off on your own.

THE BOTTOM LINE

What it all comes down to is the determination of someone to succeed. It will not matter what type of nursing specialty you decide to take up. If you have the right motivation and inspiration to succeed, then you will definitely be able to reach that six-figure salary that everyone is aiming for.

Be wise in your choices and learn as much as you can. The more experience you have, the more opportunities you can have for broadening your horizons in the world of work.

PROFESSIONAL NURSE SPOTLIGHT
6-FIGURE INCOME CAREERS IN NURSING

ARE YOU HAVING AN OUT OF MONEY EXPERIENCE?

Enlighten Up, lovely, you're standing in a long line. Nurses across the country are increasingly stating that financial debt is their number one cause of stress.

The issue isn't your job, your work, your career, your family, or your love life. The issue is your Self-Care related to the amount of "moolah" you earn and spend.

Whatever you earn, paltry or mighty, you want to increase your Self-Worth by applying golden nuggets of wisdom from the yoga of money. Let me share what I learned about growing the green from my father, and the Richest Woman in Babylon and Manhattan.

THE PROBLEM: ADDICTION TO SPENDING AND PAYING EVERYONE ELSE FIRST = BROKE GIRLS!

MONEY STRESS is the #1 PAIN POINT I hear when I give my health + wealth care remedies in talks around the country. And as a Nurse, I know and you know: STRESS KILLS! Literally!

My daddy was an Italian immigrant who came to 'America' without a pot to piss in, at age of 17 years old. He went on to become a millionaire and he taught me a thing or two about the almighty dollar.

I blew off a lot of his advice throughout "my young woman desiring absolutely everything years", still I held on tight to the basic principles.

PLUS, **my mother did not have a clue about money**, because my father controlled the purse strings, in the old fashioned Italian way in those days. Mom never learned how to handle money.

My father died when I was only nineteen **and mom ended blowing through the inheritance like a hurricane.**

I had to work hard for the rest of my life— I'm not writing to you as a coddled, spoiled rich kid living off of Daddy's money.

Now, let's move on to the **2 Top Principles of Wisdom** to fill an empty purse + nurture your soul.

PROBLEM: BROKE, HARD-WORKING NURSES

SOLUTION: PAY YOURSELF FIRST!

Impress yourself with the idea. Fill yourself with the thought. Then take whatever portion seems wise. It must not be less than one-tenth - 10 percent of all you earn. If one-tenth of all you earn is as much as you can comfortably keep, be content to keep this share...

YOU PAY EVERYONE ELSE FOR YOUR KEEP & YOUR UPKEEP; THEREFORE...YOUR NEW MANTRA + MOTTO is:

1. **"A part of all I earn is mine to keep."** Say it in the morning when you wake up. Say it at noon. Say it at night. Say it to yourself each hour of every day. Say it to yourself until the words stand out like burning letters **engraved into the software of your soul.**

2. **"Invest** in spending time learning from **conscious, wise Nurse Entrepreneurs** who nurture their nursing careers, as well as their bank accounts."

So many Nurses need a fresh infusion of money smarts. Figure it this way: eating more green makes you strong and healthy - and keeping more green makes your life abundant and wealthy. Your self-care as a nurse = wealth care + health care. Isn't it time you pay yourself first?

Annette Tersigni R.N. is an author and speaker and the founder of YogaNursing® an accredited new movement in Nursing and Health Care. The author of The Richest Woman in Babylon and Manhattan, voted an inspirational nursing book, Annette is transforming lives physically, financially and spiritually.

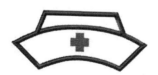

CHAPTER 29:
THE MILLIONAIRE NURSE

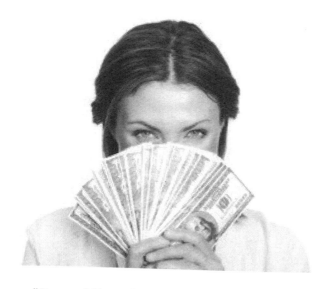

*"Do not follow where the path may lead;
go where there is not path and leave a trail."* - Anonymous

Nurse Entrepreneurs are Nurses who have been able to make use of their nursing education, skill and expertise to bring up ventures that are able to support the healthcare industry. In this regard, we are looking at Nurses who have managed to run their own companies, promote and/or establish other companies to support the healthcare system.

Some of these Nurses have also been able to come up with computerized systems, medical devices and home health products that eventually go a long way in helping the patients. There are certain skills that such Nurses possess, such as being business savvy, creative and risk takers who are able to detect a gap in the industry and possess the ability to deal with a consistent customer base.

The following are some Nurses who have not only excelled in the profession, but have also been able to venture further and become successful entrepreneurs in the process:

- Renee Baldo, BS, RN, MBA – Founder of Unlimited Potential - LLC

- Barbara Bartlein, CSP, RN, MSW – Founder of The People Pro, and has also been accredited with authoring the best seller Why Did I Marry You Anyway?

- Anthony Battaglia, RN, MS – President at Pocket Nurse®

- Vickie Milazzo – Founder of the Vickie Malazzo Institute, Legal Nurse Consultant

PROFESSIONAL NURSE SPOTLIGHT
THE MILLIONAIRE NURSE

My nursing career began as a USN Corpsman and then as a LPN while attending Nursing School to become a RN. My last role in a hospital setting was as a Charge Nurse on a Med/Surg Unit. Tired of working weekends and holidays, I began to search for different ways that I could use my nursing experience. I landed a job as a Case Manager with a major group health insurance company. It was my job to speak with the patients about their policy, what was covered and how we could determine the best way of providing their care. I was also responsible for training over 100 claim processors on the medical aspects of the claims they were processing. This job introduced me to new technology, processes and aspects of myself that I never knew before. These things combined with my nursing knowledge, primed the success that I would ultimately achieve in becoming a nurse millionaire.

I loved learning about computers and their ability to capture data that assisted healthcare professionals in analyzing healthcare outcomes. I learned about contracts, how to understand inclusions and exclusions, and how to best optimize treatment plans and resources. Of course, I loved teaching medical information to the claims processors and seeing the lights go on; I would see how they would extrapolate the information to improve their own health issues. In one way or another, I functioned in this role for several companies. I was eventually recruited by a physician to assist him in implementing his software program for a large third party administrator, Crawford & Company.

I then became the Product Manager working with software and programmers. I assisted in the creation of several offices around the country that reviewed medical bills. This also was the first time that I was in an "intrapreneurial" position by creating a new income stream within an existing company. Resigning from Crawford & Company, I was later recruited to have a central role in a start-up company that provided medical bill review services. I was responsible for operations and had 28 national offices. Each of these offices had Nurses working that were experienced in utilization review services. This company, General Review Services, merged with General Rehab Services in 1994 and later became Genex. After Genex, I was recruited to be the President of a software company called Comp Review, which was based in California. Over 1/3 of all property and casualty medical bills were processed by our software application and as we served many Fortune 500 clients. My compensation included stock options so when the company sold I became a Nurse Millionaire. I was always asked how does a Nurse end up running a multi-million dollar software company? Well, you can see the steps I took here. Today, as the President of the National Nurses in Business Association, I get to help Nurses that are interested in business on a large scale. I believe Nurses can do anything; don't be afraid to try new things!

Michelle Podlesni, RN – President of the National Nurses in Business Association. Founder and Author: *"Unconventional Nurse"*

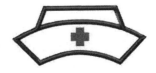

CHAPTER 30:
YOUR NEXT STEPS

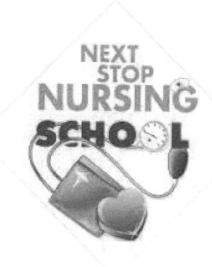

"Nurses are angels in comfortable shoes"– Unknown

With that which you have already learned in this book, you can now go on and further your career, learn and practice to become a Nurse. Even after becoming a Nurse, there is so much more for you out there.

You can still decide to diversify and become an Entrepreneur Nurse like myself, Nurse Nicole M. Brown, I ventured into teaching and writing children's books about Nursing, in a bid to explain some of the intricacies of Nursing to kids, and to encourage them to become Nurses, too, when they grow up.

Do not forget that with Nursing, your passion can take you so far, further than perhaps you would have ever imagined. As long as you are determined, nothing can stand in your way.

Remember, as a Professional Nurse, the sky is the limit for your success. After, you complete Nursing School and pass the NCLEX, you can do anything you set your mind to do.

See you at the top!!!

APPENDIX A: Q &A

WHAT MAKES NURSING A PRIME CHOICE AS A CAREER?

Nursing is a career that will allow you to serve and care for patients. It is the type of career that will give a sort of satisfaction after every day. Despite the hard journey that you will have to go through, there is also the chance that you will earn big in the long run, especially when you focus on certifications and getting more experience. This makes it a prime choice for those who want to serve their peers, and yet, earn bigger income as the years pass.

HOW DO I DETERMINE IF NURSING IS REALLY FOR ME?

Knowing whether Nursing is really a good choice for you is something that you have to think about. There may be a lot of factors that can influence your decision, but the final choice in deciding whether it is good as a career is your prerogative. You can seek guidance from Professional Nurses to find out what to expect or you can even try it out for one or two semesters to see if you like the flow of the curriculum and whether you can see yourself as a Nurse.

WHERE CAN I SEEK ADVICE WHEN I WANT TO GO TO THE BEST NURSING SCHOOL?

You can go online and search for good schools or you can also ask some Nurses in your local area for their opinions about great schools that you can go to. This will probably be your turning point so you need to do this even though it is tedious. Choosing the right school and asking about it from people who have experienced them first-hand is a valuable experience that you cannot overlook.

WHAT IS THE RELEVANCE OF PREPARING FOR NURSING SCHOOL?

Like many other courses that you want to take up, preparing to attend Nursing School is important because it will condition you about what you can expect during the next four years. You have to be in the right mindset with the proper motivation in order to be able to succeed later on. Preparation is always a must.

Being a student nurse is a demanding course. You will be pulled in all directions about the things that need to be done and you have to do your best to acclimate to all these without breaking down. To be successful, you need to know what to expect in the next years to come.

WHAT KIND OF THINGS CAN YOU DO TO PREPARE FOR IT?

You can talk with people who have taken up nursing as well and ask them about their own experiences.

Reading books and certain write ups online will also help in making you aware in terms of preparation. By knowing what the whole course entails will help you adequately prepare. This is probably all the preparation you need. Anything that needs to be learned will already be taught in the lesson so you need not worry about them before you have even enrolled.

IS THERE RELEVANCE BETWEEN THE TUITION THAT YOU HAVE TO PAY AND THE QUALITY OF EDUCATION OFFERED IN A SCHOOL?

Most well-known schools have higher tuition fees and of course, it is a given that they are able to provide quality education as well. But this is not exclusive at all. There are some training schools that have top caliber instructors, too. **You don't have to equate quality with price.**

HOW CAN I BE SURE THAT THE NURSING SCHOOL I CHOSE IS THE RIGHT ONE?

Ask around and check whether the school comes with the proper certifications. Look up their history and whether they have associations with professional Nurses. See if their students were able to tackle the licensure exams effectively. This will probably give you an accurate prediction of what you can anticipate in the future.

WHAT KIND OF CURRICULUM SHOULD I LOOK FOR?

The best curriculum is a comprehensive one. Before enrolling in a particular school, try to ask about their specific nursing programs and note the subjects that are being offered. A good school of nursing, will always have a balance of theories and practical courses so look for their counterparts at all times. You need to be able to assess them critically so that you can learn from the best and gain the right kind of knowledge that will prepare you for Nursing School.

DO I NEED SOME PRIOR QUALIFICATIONS BEFORE I CAN ATTEND A NURSING SCHOOL?

Not necessarily. But this will depend on the school that you will be attending, too. Some schools need you to take some extra credit courses while others just proceed with the entrance exam that will prepare you for admissions. All in all, the only requirement that is common to all schools is the fact that the incoming student should at least be a high school graduate.

WHAT SHOULD BE MY BIGGEST MOTIVATOR?

As a pre-nursing student who is preparing to enter this career, you need to be your biggest motivator as well. There may be instances where you were merely influenced to enter Nursing School, but in order to survive the whole two to four years and graduate, you have to understand why you are there. Your biggest motivator will be your will to end up as a Nurse. You will have to set a goal and work your way towards it in the coming years as you enter the school. There is no one that is as strong as you when it comes to motivations because so long as you hold on to that dream, you will be greatly rewarded in the long run.

DO I NEED SPECIAL CLASSES BEFORE STARTING OUT?

No. As long as you are qualified, with the right grades and have the proper years of education at your disposal, then you can enter Nursing School with no problem. Admissions will be easy as well when you pass all the needed requirements with no delay.

Those who do not have any background with nursing can be compensated by means of the subjects that are taught in the first year. You will be given the basics and backgrounds that will serve as your foundations for the upcoming years in school and in your career.

HOW LONG WILL NURSING SCHOOL LAST?

The standard for Nursing School will last two to four years. This is the basic time that needs to be completed by the students before they graduate. Every nursing professional needs to render these years in school so they can graduate and later become Registered Nurses.

WHY IS IT NECESSARY TO INVEST A LOT OF EFFORT WITH NURSING SCHOOL?

There are some speculations about what it really takes to be a Nurse, but if you are talking about investments, then the best thing you can put forward is effort. Nursing is a practical course and you will not be required to just study all the time. There are always instances when you will need to do some clinical procedures that go with it so that you learn all the basics with no compromise.

WHAT ARE MY OPTIONS AFTER GRADUATING?

If you are aspiring to be a professional Nurse, there are many options available to you. Aside from pursing further studies in nursing, you can also look up some programs that will give you some certifications about different fields. This will widen your scope in terms of becoming more than just a practicing nurse in a hospital. These certifications will become an added qualification to your growing list of skills and it will also help you out in terms of propelling your career to success after graduation.

IS IT REALLY POSSIBLE TO EARN BIGGER INCOME AS A NURSE?

Yes, as I said, you have many options with regards to careers. This also equates to various income ranges that you can avail of. Some people think that Nurses are merely limited to hospital work, but this not the case. You can even set up your own clinic later on if you have the proper qualifications. This can help you earn a greater income in the next years because instead of caring for patients, you will also get to give them some simple diagnosis and treatments.

WHAT KIND OF CAREERS CAN I CHOOSE FROM IN THE FUTURE?

Nursing is a broad choice. Although it is common knowledge that one works in the hospital, this is not always the case. You can work in the military, be affiliated with a private company, or you can go for specializations like being a Staff Nurse or as a Nurse Anesthetists. Basically, you can enter any career path as long as you make your way towards it. There may be some certifications that you need to secure, but this is all a part of the process of earning big and expanding your scope.

WHERE CAN I WORK AFTER GRADUATION?

If you want to gain more experience, then you might want to consider working at the hospital for some time after you graduated and become a registered nurse. It is a well-known fact that hospitals are abundant with cases that are unique so you can be exposed to them while you work or volunteer there. This will be your greatest advantage in the long run because not everyone is able to experience this.

These hospital situations; whether you are dealing with diseases or emergency procedures, are all integral in keeping up with the latest trends in your career. You will have the ability to handle everything flawlessly as you go through the years.

DO I NEED TO REVIEW WITH CERTIFIED CENTERS BEFORE THE NCLEX?

Yes. The NCLEX is a much needed licensure exam that you need to pass. You cannot take it for granted because it is the basis of your practice later on. It is very much advised that you seek out review centers to help you with preparing for it rather than self-study sessions. The reason for this is that you will be more equipped to deal with the examination because you know what to expect in the process.

WHY IS IT NECESSARY FOR NEW GRADUATE NURSES TO TAKE THE NCLEX?

This is one thing that you should work hard to achieve. The licensure exam is there for a reason. You cannot take it for granted because it is the basis of your practice later on. You will almost never be hired anywhere if you are someone who has not taken the exam because they will think that you lack the proper qualifications. Since you will be caring for real people in the hospital and your eventual workplace, employers will not take the chance to hire someone who is not qualified.

Is there any secret to success that I should know about when taking Nursing as a course and eventual career?

The secret to success in Nursing lies within you. Much like any other course that you decide to take in college, it will require motivation and perseverance. You have to keep your eyes on the prize – graduation, and then work your way from there. This will be your goal and your journey towards it will be your keys to success in school and in your eventual career. This course is a hard one and you have to be practical in all approaches to it in order to succeed. You cannot bow down to the demands and give up in the middle.

APPENDIX B

The Steps to become a Professional Nurse

If you are applying to become a Registered Nurse (RN), you do not have a degree in Nursing. Application to nursing schools is usually done on a rolling basis, which means that the students are free to apply for summer, fall or spring semesters and in most cases may have to write an essay to be considered.

You will need to have attained a GPA of at least a 3.0 to be considered; each school's GPA requirements can vary. The process to complete the nursing school pre-requisites may take 1 to 2 years to complete.

The 10 steps to becoming a Professional Nurse:

1. Find a Professional Nursing School

2. Meet with the Advisors

3. Apply for admission

4. Complete Prerequisites

5. Receive Admissions Decision

6. Complete FAFSA form

7. Attend Nursing School

8. Complete Clinical Rotations

9. Graduate/Apply for NCLEX

10. Pass NCLEX

APPENDIX C: RECOURSES

WEBSITE RESOURCES FOR FUTURE NURSING STUDENTS

All Nurses (www.AllNurses.com) – A platform that allows new, aspiring and existing Nurses to interact with one another. There are more than 800,000 Nurses in the database who share ideas on this forum.

Educational Portal– An information hub that allows future Nurses and current Nurses the various types of nursing education available to succeed as a Nurse.

Explore Health Careers (www.ExploreHealthCareers.Org) – A network that provides all the information you need on careers in health, Nursing in particular:

Forensic Nurse (www.ForensicNurses.Org) – if you have been keen on becoming a Forensic Nurse this is the website for you, with articles, news and all kinds of information that you need

Nurse Zone (www.NurseZone.com) – There are a lot of journals and resources that can guide you as a nurse here.

Nurse.com (www.Nurse.com) – This is a website that is dedicated to Nursing, with all information on almost all elements of Nursing, from community to education.

Nursing World (www.NursingWorld.org) – Provides all the latest news in the world of Nursing.

NLM Gateway (http://gateway.nlm.nih.gov/) – provides all the access you need to government information on health subjects.

The American Nurses Association (www.NursingWorld.org)

– A professional organization that represents the interests of more than 3 million Nurses registered within the profession.

BOOK RESOURCES FOR FUTURE STUDENT NURSES

Keys to Nursing Success (Katz, Carter, Bishop & Kravits,

2009) - A guide to help nursing students realize needed change and improve their lives.

Test Success (Nugent & Vitale, 2008) – This book is designed to help the beginning nursing students to take and pass nursing school tests successfully.

ABOUT THE AUTHOR

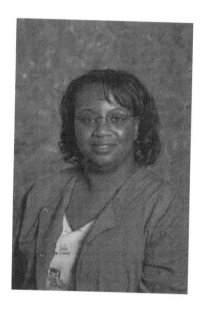

Nicole M. Brown, MSN, RN (Doctoral Candidate)

I am a Professional Nurse.

When I was young and in high school, I also did not know what course to take so I brainstormed a lot. I thought I wanted to be a doctor or a lawyer, like my other family members. I was discouraged from becoming a nurse. I was told nurses did not make enough money and they worked the hardest in the hospital. I soon joined the US Army Reserves as a Chaplain's Assistant to pay for college and was accepted into a Pre-med program. I found myself deployed to Germany for Operation Desert Storm.

Upon returning from Germany, I decide that Pre-med and Med School were too long to be dependent financial on my family. I decide to go to Nursing School because I wanted to be financially independent.

So, I started my journey to pursue a Professional Nursing degree.

I found my calling. I felt like I have found my purpose in life.

From then and there, the rest was history. This was how I started my life's chapter in becoming a Professional Nurse.

Let me relay to you my experience from being a student to eventual a nursing professional. I was not by any means a skillful person. But I'd like to believe that my greatest advantage was my passion for work. Nursing was not just something that I enrolled in because I was forced to do so. It was really what I wanted and this realization has been my principle that led me to finish school, pass the NCLEX, and become a professional Nurse.

I looked for the best school that I could find and found out that taking up Nursing is not something that can be done on a whim. A lot of people think that just because it entails fewer requirements compared to a doctor, then it is easier. But this is not the case.

In fact, we have worked hard before we finally became what we are now.

The journey to becoming a Professional Nurse is a hard road that not everyone can survive.

I started out with a lot of people as classmates, but only a few were really able to stand the demands as we breezed through the semesters. Some of them declared that Nursing was not for them. Others claimed that they could not handle the stress because of too many lessons and memorizations that needed to be absorbed.

As a student, there were times that the subjects were hard while the instructors were even harder to understand. It gave large amounts of stress to everyone. It was a hard battle, indeed.

I admit that there were also times when I wanted to quit as well. Some days were just so bad that I wanted to drop everything and suddenly take up Fine Arts or something. But then again, I had a goal in mind and I promised myself that no matter what happened or what might come my way, I will stick to that goal.

I wanted to be a Professional Nurse.

After a bit of calming down and some reflection on my part, I always came to the conclusion that Fine Arts would not do it for me. I had my calling and I will go for it!

Now I am not here to brag about the hardships that I have withstood in Nursing School. I pointed them out because it is necessary for all of you to understand at least a part of what I went through. I am here today in order to share a more enlightened fact, and that is how to survive in Nursing School.

It all comes down to three things basically and you'd be surprised at how simple it may seem.

I succeeded and survived school because of Belief, Confidence, and Perseverance.

Let's start off with the first one. There was once a time when I only imagined myself in a white uniform while caring for ailing patients. But look, here I am now, a professional. Anyone successful has once aspired to become what he or she is now. It just takes a little belief on your part.

As they say, if you can imagine it, then there is nothing that can stand in your way of achieving it. If you can see yourself as a Nurse, then go for it! Do not be discouraged. You have your belief, so why not push and push until you finally have it in your grasp.

Believe in your teachers, believe in the subjects that you take and most of all, believe in yourself. This is the first step in becoming a great and successful student nurse.

Next, there is confidence.

A lot of people make mistakes during school and nursing students are no exception. Those who are taking this course will probably undergo a whole new wave of mistakes and they will be reprimanded for it. But my advice for them is to not give up. Be confident. Sure, you have made a mistake now, but there is always next time and you can do it better. You will be more confident by then.

Some would say that this kind of self-assurance is not really needed, but this is not the case. You don't have to be boastful, just have faith in yourself because you know what you are doing. Confidence is a great armor against all adversities.

Even if you are afraid to perform a procedure for the first time, don't let it get to you. Admit to being nervous, but do your best all the same.

Let it become a mantra of sorts for you. Be confident! Lastly, there is perseverance.

Perhaps, among the three, I'd like to believe this is the most important one. I have relayed to you my experiences about Nursing School and you might have noticed that they were hard ones. We didn't have it easy. Anyone who is aspiring to be a future Nurse will be subjected to all of these difficulties. You will have to juggle time, priorities, tasks, and many other factors in your life during school.

There will be days when you just want to lie down and cry because everything might turn out to be too much. And amidst all of this, you will need your most powerful weapon, and that is perseverance.

Perseverance is your ability to stand up again and again despite failures and discouragements. There are a lot of people who lose their morale because they did not do well with certain subjects. Eventually, they find themselves giving up. Do not be one of these people.

Take heed that as long as you persevere, then you will always have a greater potential to succeed. This is your chance to be a better person as a student nurse. It will be hard, yes, but you cannot allow yourself to be deterred by common mistakes. This might eventually become your biggest regret.

Giving up is not a part of being successful. Sometimes your body might not be able to make it anymore despite your mind still being active and ready. These two will clash, but once again, persevere.

When your professor calls you out on a mistake, persevere.

When other students feel like giving up, don't emulate them. Take a stand and persevere.

After you have achieved your goal of graduating, it doesn't stop there. You have to go through the licensure exams before you can become a professional. You will still need these three values. Don't throw them away just because you have finished school. They are applicable to all sectors of your life, as well, so learn well and do better.

Your licensure exams will be another hard journey that you have to tackle. It's a draining experience, but it is also something worth fighting for. When you pass and become a Nurse with the attachment of RN in your name, then there is no greater feeling.

I know because I have gone through it myself. Suddenly, all those hardships were nothing. And at that time, I was at my proudest moment and on my highest peak. I was literally on top of the world for a moment when the results came out. You'll probably feel that too when that time comes.

From then on, the rest was history. I became a Professional Nurse and achieved my dream. Life is good!

I have imparted to you my journey through Nursing School. It may not have been the perfect path filled with leisurely walks, but rest assured that there will come a time when it will all be worth it.

I am proud to be a Nurse. And for all of you who are aspiring to be the same thing, I hope that you also take into consideration what I have stated here.

The journey is quite tedious and rocky, but as long as you have the proper motivation, mindset, and beliefs, you will be able to survive whatever Nursing School or your career path may throw at you. Just don't give up. Take one-step forward each day, and before you know it, you will have it!

HAPPY NURSING EVERYONE!!!!

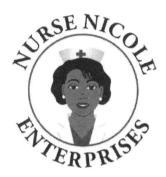

Nicole M. Brown, MSN, RN is the Founder of Nurse Nicole Enterprises, which develops children's books, animated DVD and dolls to explain nursing to children in a fun and creative way. Bulk orders are available! Go to http://nursingsuccesscollege.com/gift-and-resource-shop

Books: The Adventures of Nurse Nicole; N is for Nurse, Wash Your Hands & My Body

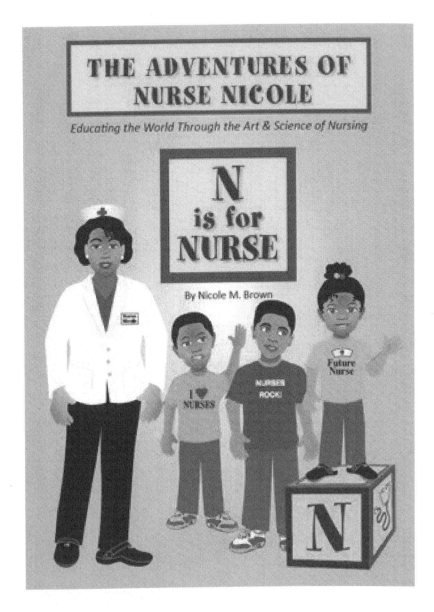

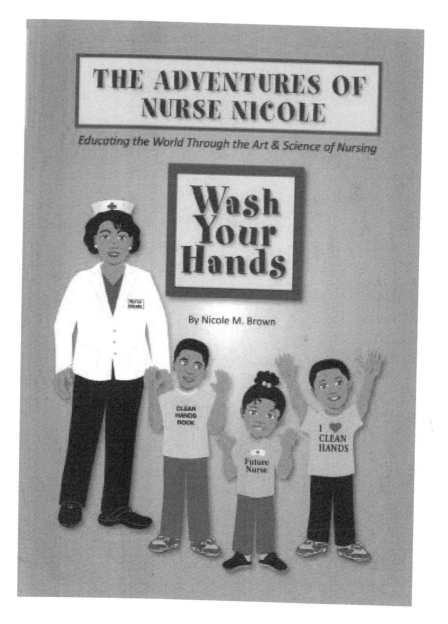

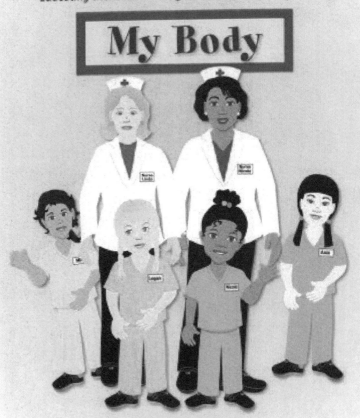

By Nicole M. Brown

DVD: BATTLE OF THE GERMS

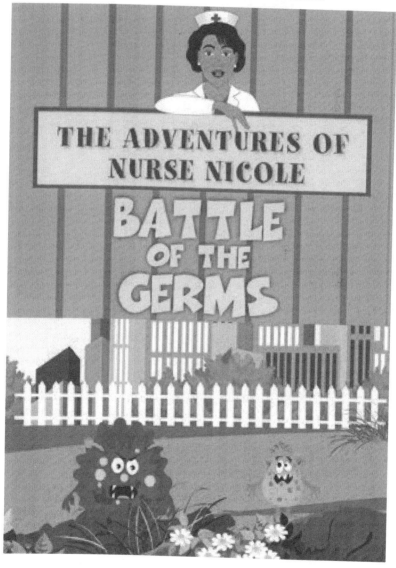

DOLLS: NURSE LINDA & NURSE NICOLE

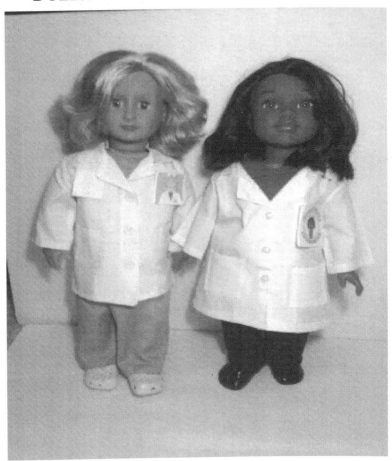

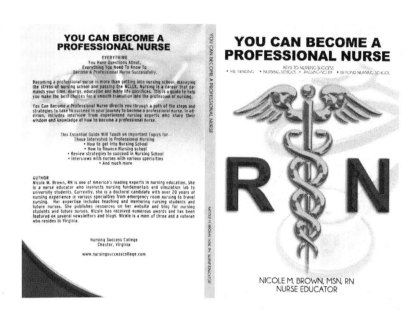

Bring "You Can Become a Professional Nurse"
to your organization!

Bring "You Can Become a Professional Nurse" to your organization!

In today's world, there is a need to increase the population of RN's to improve the outcomes of healthcare from the bedside to the boardroom.

Nursing and healthcare leaders often dream of having a school available to teach people about the profession of nursing. Heavy focus is on providing knowledge of various careers in the field of nursing. Nursing students are required to spend long hours preparing for class and studying; Nursing Success College provides them with resources to transition to becoming an organized nursing student.

How can future nursing students or current nursing students stay engaged in nursing school and keep on task with their study schedules?

If you are a nurse or healthcare leader who cares about the well-being of future or student nurses, but feels guilty about the lack of time, capital or resources available – I am here to help!!!

Do not spend another sleepless night trying to figure out how to "fix" your nursing students to improve retention and grades; I have an easy, convenient and cost effective answer for you.

As a motivational speaker, I can provide:

- Brief on-the-go self-care touches for future or student nurses in the form of in-services, lunch-and-learn, or virtual webinars.

- More formal, yet highly engaging and inspirational presentations in the form of keynote speeches and convention programs talks.

- Interactive, hands-on training in the form of half day seminars, full day workshops, or extended in person retreats.

Contact me to have a program started for your organization today!!!!

The workbook is available as a resource and guide with this book. In addition, CD's and CEU's are coming soon!!!

Contact: Nicole M. Brown, MSN, RN

Phone (863) 221-1778

info@nursingsuccesscollege.com

Website: http://nursingsuccesscollege.com/

Facebook: https://www.facebook.com/NurseNicoleMBrown

Twitter: https://twitter.com/authornursenmb

Linked In: www.linkin.com/pub/nicole-m-brown/55/4a4/748/

Made in the USA
San Bernardino, CA
15 October 2017